# CLINICAL DECISION LEVELS FOR LAB TESTS

# CLINICAL DECISION LEVELS FOR LAB TESTS

## Bernard E. Statland, MD, PhD

Director, Department of Laboratory Medicine
University Hospital, Boston
Professor of Pathology and Medicine
Boston University Medical School

Medical Economics Books
Oradell, New Jersey 07649

**Library of Congress Cataloging in Publication Data**

Statland, Bernard E.
  Clinical decision levels for lab tests.

  Includes index.
  1. Diagnosis, Laboratory—Decision making.  I. Title.
[DNLM: 1. Diagnosis, Laboratory. 2. Decision making.
QY4 S797c]
RB37.S695 1983      616.07′56      83-8342
ISBN 0-87489-301-1


Cover design by William Kuhn

ISBN 0-87489-301-1

Medical Economics Company Inc.
Oradell, New Jersey 07649

Printed in the United States of America

*To Ellis Benson, for first
introducing me to the challenges
and opportunities of laboratory
medicine*

*And to Alexandra, Eli, and Beverly,
in deep appreciation for their
understanding and support*

# CONTENTS

# FOREWORD

## John W. Burnside, M.D.

Clinical decision making is a complicated process. The astute physician relies on several sources of information in order to determine: (a) Is this patient sick? (b) If yes, what is the nature of the condition? (c) How serious is the condition? (d) How quickly must I act?

Among the means available to assist in this process, the modern clinical laboratory is one that has contributed greatly to our clinical decision-making abilities. Yet, like any sophisticated instrument, the clinical laboratory must be understood before it can be used effectively. We physicians frequently misuse the laboratory. The costs of misuse—in terms of dollars, false positives, false negatives, repeated tests, and anxieties from misinformation—are very high.

In this text, Dr. Bernard Statland reminds us of some of the complexities involved in establishing normal values, the variables that affect test outcomes, and the delineation of confidence limits. In lucid detail, he shows how confidence limits vary, depending on whether we wish to include or exclude a disease as a possibility.

The history and physical examination are the first steps applied in the sequential analysis of a patient's problems. From the responses and findings, the differential diagnosis is established. This is merely a list of probabilities, but it represents the critical first step. Students of Bayes's theorem understand that the diagnostic accuracy of a test is critically related to the prevalence of the suspected condition in the test population. Even a test that is 95 percent sensitive and 95 percent specific is diagnostic only when the likelihood of that condition is high. Random screening can never replace this judgment.

The first portion of this volume is a text and the second a reference. The first portion is required reading for all who hope to make the most of their abilities in using a clinical laboratory. The reference section is a valuable reminder of the nature of aberrations that can lead to abnormal laboratory results, and includes all those unusual entities that in our haste we may forget.

This slim volume is a gem that deserves to be a constant companion.

John W. Burnside, M.D.
Professor of Medicine and Chief, Division of Internal
    Medicine
Milton S. Hershey Medical Center
Pennsylvania State University College of Medicine
Hershey, Pennsylvania

# FOREWORD

## Robert J. Fitzgibbon

Once in a great while, an author is able to look at existing data in a different way and translate them into terms that have vastly greater usefulness and application. That is what Bernard Statland has achieved in this book with his concept of decision levels.

As he explains so lucidly in Part One, there are serious drawbacks in using reference values in clinical decision making. Decision levels, on the other hand, overcome this inadequacy by pinpointing thresholds above or below which a particular action is recommended.

The heart of the book—indeed, the bulk of it—is Part Two, which provides decision levels for 71 commonly tested analytes. The analytes are grouped into seven categories: electrolytes, metabolites, proteins and enzymes, hormones, hematology tests, miscellaneous tests, and drug assays. For each analyte, the author presents the reference interval, causes of increased and decreased values, and decision levels along with recommended actions or considerations for each level. To facilitate using this manual, it was designed so that the information for each analyte is presented on two facing pages. The design also took into consideration the likelihood that readers will have occasion to enter their own notes.

Dr. Statland is one of the nation's most brilliant young clinical pathologists. He is director of laboratory medicine and professor of pathology and medicine at Boston University Medical Center. In addition to reference values, his areas of investigative interest range from enzyme determinations to fetal maturity testing to cancer tumor markers.

Dr. Statland's first published article on decision levels appeared in *Diagnostic Medicine*. He is also familiar to readers of *MLO* as the editor of that journal's popular Tips on Technology department.

This manual is extraordinary in that clinicians as well as laboratorians can profitably read and use it. It can guide the clinical decision making of the former and enhance the consultative role of the latter.

Robert J. Fitzgibbon
Editorial Director
*MLO, Diagnostic Medicine, CLR*

# PUBLISHER'S NOTES

Bernard E. Statland, M.D., Ph.D., is director of the Department of Laboratory Medicine, University Hospital, Boston, and professor in Boston University Medical School's Departments of Pathology and Medicine.

Dr. Statland has published numerous articles and abstracts and has contributed chapters to several scholarly books, among them the 16th edition of *Todd-Sanford-Davidsohn Clinical Diagnosis and Management by Laboratory Methods*. He was an assistant editor of that work, responsible for the section on clinical chemistry.

This book is graced with two forewords. John W. Burnside, M.D., who wrote the first foreword, is professor of medicine, Pennsylvania State University College of Medicine, and chief, Division of Internal Medicine, Milton S. Hershey Medical Center, Hershey, Pa. He is the author of the 16th edition of *Physical Diagnosis: An Introduction to Clinical Medicine*.

Robert J. Fitzgibbon, author of the second foreword, is editorial director of *MLO, Diagnostic Medicine*, and *CLR*. He is the editor also of *Legal Guidelines for the Clinical Laboratory*, published in 1981 by Medical Economics Books.

# INTRODUCTION

Since the 1950s, there has been an unprecedented growth in the number of laboratory tests available to physicians and in the total number of tests physicians are ordering. It has become almost impossible, even for the specialist in laboratory medicine, to be aware of all of the clinical indications for these tests, the appropriate normal — or reference — intervals, and the best use of these tests for decision making.

It's my intention in this manual to dispel some of the mystery that has surrounded the concept of normal values, to promote the use of the term decision level to refer to a point at which laboratory values take on a certain relevance for patient management, and to identify decision levels for specific actions. The manual contains significant decision levels for 71 commonly ordered laboratory tests. Use of these decision levels should result in more efficient patient management.

The book is divided into two parts. The first — Chapters 1 to 3 — presents the development of decision levels in laboratory testing. It begins with a discussion of normal, or reference, values, proceeds with the definition of decision levels, and then concludes with an explanation of how to use the information presented in this manual. The second part deals with the laboratory measurements of specific analytes, including reference values for each analyte and therapeutic intervals for drug assays, the causes of increased or decreased values, and decision levels with appropriate guidelines for action. Finally, there is an alphabetical list of the 71 analytes included in this book.

Feel free to modify reference values according to your own locally derived values, add additional causes of increased or decreased results, and even add or delete various decision levels as the class of patients you treat may dictate. This manual is meant to be a working clinical tool, not a didactic textbook.

I've intended this book also to be an aid to clinical judgment, not a substitute for it. Use these decision levels as they are given here or according to your modifications, but don't rely so heavily on them that you fail to perceive important nuances in the clinical presentation.

# PART

## ONE

# The Development of Decision Levels in Laboratory Testing

# CHAPTER

# 1      Reference Values

Almost all texts in laboratory medicine as well as most report forms have a suggested normal range associated with each laboratory test. For example, the most recent edition of *Todd-Sanford-Davidsohn Clinical Diagnosis and Management by Laboratory Methods* lists the normal range for serum bilirubin as 0.1–1.2 mg/dl (1.7–20.5 $\mu$mol/L).

How did we come to use the term normal value or the term reference interval? Obviously, the major purpose is to compare an individual lab result with some standard. The standard is generally derived from values obtained from healthy subjects and usually is the computed middle 95 percent of such results. Using our example for serum bilirubin, we can assume that 0.1–1.2 mg/dl represents the interval that encompasses 95 percent of values obtained from healthy subjects. This is computed by means of either a parametric or a nonparametric approach.

The *parametric approach* is based on an assumption that the values obtained from healthy subjects follow a Gaussian distribution, or a normal distribution as it is also called. The Gaussian distribution is such that if one were to determine the mean and standard deviation of the values, then the mean minus two standard deviations and the mean plus two standard deviations would encompass approximately 95 percent of the values in a given population.

The *nonparametric approach* makes no assumptions pertaining to the distribution of values. One first obtains a series of results in a population of healthy subjects. The results are listed in increasing or decreasing order. The 2.5 percentile value and the 97.5 percentile value are determined. These values will then contain the middle 95 percent interval.

It so happens that the parametric approach can be justifiably applied to about 50 percent of lab tests. For the remaining tests, a transformation of the values may be necessary to normalize the distribution. Then the mean and standard deviations are calculated. When the transformation is not successful in normalizing the distribution, the nonparametric approach should be used. In the serum bilirubin example presented above, the values do not conform to the idealized Gaussian distribution. The reference limits of 0.1 and 1.2 were determined with a nonparametric approach.

## Reference Values vs. Normal Values

In 1967, Grasbeck and Saris* proposed the term reference values as an alternative to normal values. They contended that the adjective normal was too misleading. Normal could theoretically refer to the average value, the ideal value, the type of distribution (Gaussian), or to health. The term reference value, on the other hand, implies that the values of a patient are to be referred to a comparable set of values obtained from similar subjects — similar regarding age, sex, and other demographic characteristics.

Over the past few years, various national and international committees have attempted to resolve controversies related to the issue of reference values. A number of recommendations have resulted from such deliberations. It's now generally agreed that the following definitions are in order:

▶ **A reference population:** the population on whom reference values are obtained.

▶ **Reference values:** a series of values obtained from a reference population, for example, a serum bilirubin result from each of a number of subjects of the reference population.

▶ **Reference interval:** a range of values obtained from the reference value set. Usually this interval is the middle 95 percent of all reference values. Thus, the lower reference limit is the 2.5 percentile while the upper reference limit is the 97.5 percentile.

---

*Grasbeck R and Saris NE. Establishment and use of normal values. *Scand J Clin Lab Invest* 24 (supplement 110):62, 1969.

## How Reference Values Are Produced

There are a number of steps involved in producing reference values. They include the following:
- ► A sample of a population is selected.
- ► Each member of the sample is subjected to specimen collection and the specimen is processed in the usual manner.
- ► The specimen is assayed for the analyte(s) of interest.
- ► Using various statistical and mathematical approaches, the data are reduced so as to define a (95 percent) reference interval.

**Selection of subjects.** Obviously, if one wishes to produce reference intervals for a particular demographic group, it would be inappropriate to select subjects from a different population. For example, reference values to be used for pediatric patients should not be derived from geriatric subjects. Thus, it's critical to be aware of the various demographic considerations that affect reference values. To continue the example, pediatric reference values differ from adult values for such analytes as alkaline phosphatase (higher), inorganic phosphorus (higher), and creatinine (lower). Most often, due to convenience, reference values are based upon results obtained from subjects working in a clinical laboratory, from medical students, or from healthy blood donors. Although these subjects can serve as a reference population, their values may not always be appropriate for evaluating the results from a sick patient who is hospitalized, who may be elderly, and who may be on various medications.

**Obtaining the specimen and processing it.** The conditions in which the specimen from a patient is collected may dramatically affect the resultant value. The critical circumstances include:
- ► prior physical activity,
- ► posture of the subject,
- ► previous ethanol ingestion,
- ► prior drug ingestion,
- ► previous diet,
- ► smoking history,
- ► tourniquet application time, and
- ► time of day when the specimen was obtained.

A few examples may illustrate the significance of the circumstances of specimen collection. *Prior physical exercise* can produce increased enzyme values in muscle, for example, creatine kinase, SGOT, and LDH. Going from the supine to the standing *posture* increases values in the nonfilterable substances in blood such as albumin, total protein, and protein-bound substances. *Ethanol ingestion* results in both short- and long-term changes. Short-term changes include increased serum urate and plasma lactate, and decreased plasma glucose. Long-term changes—more than two days after ingestion—include increased serum gamma glutamyl transferase, HDL cholesterol, and triglycerides. With regard to *prior food intake*, a meal high in fat prior to specimen collection, for example, causes changes due both to methodologic as well as physiologic factors. The methodologic problems are based on the fact that resultant lipemia increases the turbidity of the solution, which affects laboratory measurement if the value depends on absorbance at the same wavelength. Physiologic changes include increased alkaline phosphatase occurring after a fatty meal.

In addition to the above factors, the preparation of the specimen may also affect laboratory results, for example, contamination with anticoagulants and preservatives, the production of serum or plasma from the venipuncture tube, the preparation of a urine aliquot from a urine collection, the stability or instability of analytes upon storage, the thawing and freezing of a specimen, and evaporation-induced errors. It is important that the preparation of the specimen obtained from the reference population be similar to that obtained from the clinical population.

**Analytical procedure.** Once the subjects from whom reference values are to be produced have been chosen and the specimens have been obtained and processed, the samples are analyzed. The analytical procedure is fraught with the potential for error. The errors or variations are of two general types, random error and systematic error.

*Random error* refers to the imprecision or variability of the assay itself. Such variability can never be completely avoided. It relates to variability in fluid dispensing, the imprecision of the electrical-optical aspects of the instrument itself, and the variations that may occur with any other step in the analysis. The imprecision may be greater from day to day or batch to batch than it is within a day or within a batch. Since the variation of the reference specimens should be similar in magnitude and type to the variation in the specimens taken from the clinical population, the reference values should be produced over a number of days or a number of batches.

*Systematic error (bias)* should be the same for the assays determined on the reference population as it is for the clinical population. Thus, the same type of reagent, the same instrument, and exactly the same method should be used for both cases. The presence of a systematic error is apparent when a set of results does not correspond to that obtained in a study done with a definitive method. Such information is usually available through a laboratory's proficiency studies.

**Data reduction.** Once the results on the reference population are available, the reference interval can be computed. The distribution of values is first analyzed to see if it corresponds to the Gaussian, or normal, distribution. If so, the mean and the standard deviation are determined. The middle 95 percent interval is then defined as $\bar{x} - 2SD$, $\bar{x} + 2SD$ ($\bar{x}$ is the mean, and SD the standard deviation).

As suggested earlier, if the values do not correspond to the Gaussian distribution, they can be transformed into values that may correspond to it. The transformation may be logarithmic or a square root transformation, for example. The transformed values are then examined to see if *they* correspond to the Gaussian distribution. If not, the nonparametric approach discussed above is used to determine the middle 95 percent interval.

## The Significance of the Reference Interval

When a value derived from a patient is outside the reference limits, you can make only a general inference—that is, that there is a strong probability that the patient is not a member of the theoretical group from which the sample population was selected. If a patient is outside the reference interval, we can conclude that one of the following statements is true:
- ▶ The patient is sick.
- ▶ The patient is well, but is a statistical outlier.
- ▶ The patient is well, but is demographically different from the reference population.

► The patient is well, but the preparation of the specimen was different from that of the reference population.

► The patient is well, but he engaged in activities prior to specimen collection that caused his values to be outside the reference limits.

Unfortunately, clinicians tend to rely upon a reference interval to answer the question "Is the patient ill?" A patient could be ill, yet a value for a particular analyte might be within the reference interval. Conversely, the patient could be well but have a value outside the reference limit. The reason reference values can be somewhat misleading is that the alternative question is not asked. The alternative question is: "What should we conclude when the value is outside the reference limit?" We look at this problem more explicitly in the next chapter.

# CHAPTER

# 2 Decision Levels

There are many reasons to order laboratory tests—some legitimate and some not so legitimate; the principal appropriate ones are these four: to detect, to confirm, to classify, and to monitor.

In addition to these major reasons, there also are some less proper, but nonetheless compelling, reasons to do laboratory measurements.

They include:
► medical curiosity,
► fear of malpractice suits,
► compliance with attending physician's demands,
► response to patient's wishes, and
► financial considerations.

If a laboratory measurement is to be of any value, it must affect the management of a patient. If the management of a patient will not change due to a laboratory result, the decision to order such a laboratory test must be questioned. There are three major patient-management actions that could result from laboratory testing:
► changing the therapeutic regimen on a patient,
► ordering additional diagnostic tests, and
► sharing prognostic information with a patient or a patient's family.

## Reference Intervals and Decision Making

Many physicians are tempted to rely heavily upon reference limits in their clinical decision making. Unfortunately, reference limits are insufficient for this task. You cannot necessarily deduce a clinical

**Figure 1**

*Theoretical distribution of subjects for a laboratory measurement*

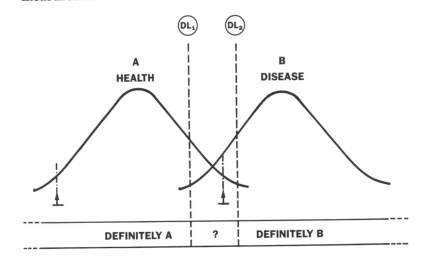

decision simply on the basis of whether a lab result is outside a particular reference interval.

Figure 1 presents the theoretical distribution of two groups of subjects for a particular laboratory measurement. Group A is the group of individuals who are in a state of good health. The reference interval is defined by the two arrows. Group B is a group of individuals with a particular illness. The critical issue is whether a subject is a member of group B, the members of which, we assume, would benefit from therapy. Whether the individual is within or outside the reference limit for healthy subjects is academic. It's more relevant to ask whether a particular patient is a member of a group for which therapy will make a difference.

The limiting value, the other side of which membership in a group of subjects suffering from a particular disease can be excluded, is designated $DL_1$. There is another limiting value. That value is designated $DL_2$, a value on one side of which all subjects must be members of group B. In that case, therapy could be invoked, depending upon its side effects and efficacy.

These two limiting values can also be termed decision levels. The first decision level is the *point of exclusion*. The second decision

## Figure 2

*Distribution of subjects for a theoretical enzyme test*

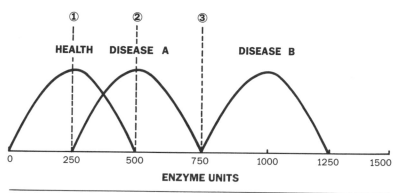

Circled numbers indicate decision levels.

level is the *point of confirmation.* An alternative term for point of exclusion is point of detection. All subjects who are members of group B have values to the right of the point of detection.

It should be obvious that decision levels—practical guideposts for clinical decision making—may be distinct from reference limits. In Figure 1, the left reference limit is far removed from the first decision level, and, though the right reference limit is more closely related to the point of exclusion, it is not identical to it.

## Definition of Decision Levels

The term decision level, which I use throughout this book, was first introduced by Barnett in 1968.* A decision level is a threshold value above which or below which a particular management action is recommended. Usually, the values assigned to decision levels are those limiting values that are used to exclude or confirm membership in a particular clinical class or to warn of significant physiologic effects that are likely to occur when a particular analyte, which is usually held in homeostatic control, reaches that value.

Figure 2 illustrates such a relationship between decision levels and reference limits for a theoretical test involving a new enzyme.

*Barnett RN. Medical significance of laboratory results. *Am J Clin Pathol* 50:671-676, 1968.

## Figure 3

*Calcium*

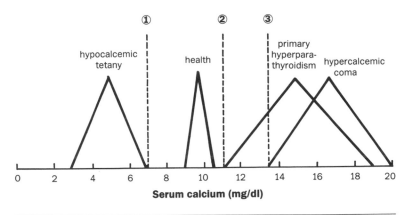

Circled numbers indicate decision levels.

| REFERENCE INTERVAL | LEVEL 1 | LEVEL 2 | LEVEL 3 |
|---|---|---|---|
| 9.0–10.6 mg/dl | 7.0 mg/dl | 11.0 mg/dl | 13.5 mg/dl |
| (2.25–2.65 mmol/L) | (1.75 mmol/L) | (2.75 mmol/L) | (3.4 mmol/L) |

One of the decision levels for the test is 500 enzyme units. This decision level is, in fact, the same value as the upper reference limit determined for the healthy subjects. The other two decision levels (250 and 750 units), however, do not coincide with either reference limit. A value of 1000 or one of 1200 results in the same action, because both values exceed the 750 decision level.

Figures 3 to 6 show relationships between reference limits and decision levels for four laboratory tests. There are four clinical classes associated with serum calcium levels (Figure 3). The 95 percent interval representing healthy adults is defined by the values 9.0 mg/dl and 10.6 mg/dl.

The values observed in hypocalcemic tetany, which is associated with a high risk of convulsions, range from 3 mg/dl to 7 mg/dl. Because it is so important to detect all such patients, one decision level is set at 7 mg/dl. Whenever a serum calcium value is below 7 mg/dl, additional diagnostic tests should be done to assess the possibility of the patient's going into tetany. Preventive measures may also be necessary.

## Figure 4

*Albumin*

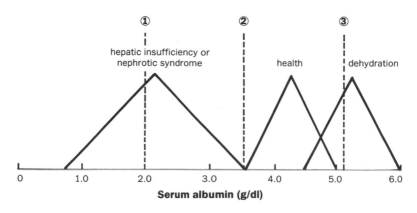

Circled numbers indicate decision levels.

| REFERENCE INTERVAL | LEVEL 1 | LEVEL 2 | LEVEL 3 |
|---|---|---|---|
| 3.5–5.0 g/dl | 2.0 g/dl | 3.5 g/dl | 5.2 g/dl |
| (35–50 g/L) | (20 g/L) | (35 g/L) | (52 g/L) |

The lower limit of the range of values observed in primary hyperparathyroidism is 11 mg/dl and is defined as the second decision level. Primary hyperparathyroidism should be tested and ruled out by appropriate laboratory measurements. Many subjects suffering from this disorder have renal stones, hypertension, or duodenal ulcers.

The fourth clinical class is defined by values seen in hypercalcemic coma. Patients in this group must be identified without delay, and so the third decision level is set at 13.5 mg/dl, the low value for this clinical class.

It is clear from the figure that two of the three decision levels are not close to the reference limits.

There are three clinical classes associated with serum albumin levels (Figure 4). One decision level is set at 3.5 g/dl to detect all instances of low serum albumin values.

The decision level of 5.2 g/dl is somewhat higher than the upper reference limit. This avoids the problem of many false positives.

**Figure 5**

*Glucose*

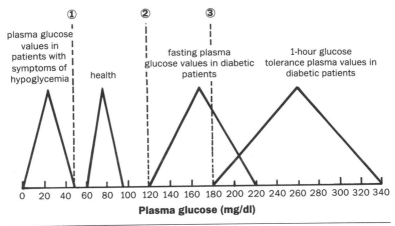

Circled numbers indicate decision levels.

| REFERENCE INTERVAL | LEVEL 1 | LEVEL 2 | LEVEL 3 |
|---|---|---|---|
| 60–95 mg/dl | 45 mg/dl | 120 mg/dl | 180 mg/dl |
| (3.33–5.28 mmol/L) | (2.5 mmol/L) | (6.6 mmol/L) | (10.0 mmol/L) |

The decision level at 2.0 g/dl is set there because patients who have liver disease and albumin levels below 2.0 g/dl have a very grave prognosis.

Four groups are associated with plasma glucose levels (Figure 5). One of them that demands attention is composed of patients who have hypoglycemia-associated symptoms. The range of values for this class is 0 to 45 mg/dl. Because all members of this group should be identified, one decision level is 45 mg/dl.

Two clinical classes group glucose values in diabetic patients. One is fasting plasma glucose values and the other includes the glucose tolerance test value at one hour. Since both classes need to be identified, the threshold values are at the lower ends of these two ranges. The decision levels are 120 mg/dl and 180 mg/dl, respectively. There could also be additional decision levels at the upper end of the scale to identify patients having nonketotic hyperglycemic coma.

Three clinical classes are associated with specific ranges of serum ALT (SGPT) levels (Figure 6). The reference range for

## Figure 6

*Alanine aminotransferase (ALT, SGPT)*

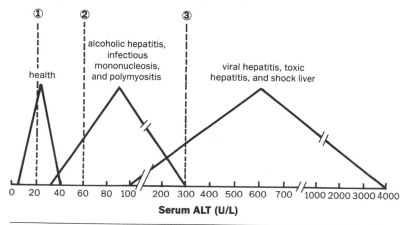

Circled numbers indicate decision levels.

| REFERENCE INTERVAL | LEVEL 1 | LEVEL 2 | LEVEL 3 |
|---|---|---|---|
| 5–40 U/L at 37°C | 20 U/L | 60 U/L | 300 U/L |

healthy subjects is 5 to 40 U/L. These values are for assays performed at 37°C.

Increased values of ALT usually occur in conjunction with hepatocellular destruction, and two groups can be identified. The group with profound increases in ALT consists of patients who have massive liver destruction as a result of viral hepatitis, toxic hepatitis, or shock liver (hypoperfused liver). The other group of values is associated with mild hepatocellular destruction. Such cases include alcoholic hepatitis and infectious mononucleosis.

The three decision levels are 20 U/L, 60 U/L, and 300 U/L. The value of 300 U/L discriminates between two types of hepatocellular destruction; all values above this level lead to the assumption of profound hepatocellular destruction.

The second decision level is 60 U/L—somewhat greater than the upper reference limit. This higher limit avoids unnecessary classification of patients as having hepatocellular destruction. Many patients with values between 40 and 60 U/L do not have demonstrable hepatocellular destruction. It may be difficult to identify causes for such elevations in ALT. Increased ALT often occurs with obesity in an otherwise healthy subject.

The decision level of 20 U/L is an exclusion threshold. All values below this level lead to a rejection of the hypothesis that the patient suffers from hepatocellular destruction. The only exception is profound massive hepatocellular insufficiency, but this entity can certainly be identified clinically.

# CHAPTER

## 3    How to Use This Manual

The heart of this manual is the presentation of decision levels for 71 laboratory tests. Each analyte is explicitly defined in terms of a suggested reference interval, a list of commonly occurring causes for increased as well as for decreased values, and then a number of proposed decision levels. Along with each decision level is a suggested course of action to follow when the result is either above or below that threshold.

The 71 analytes are divided into seven categories: electrolytes, metabolites, proteins and enzymes, hormones, hematology-related tests, miscellaneous tests, and drugs. For each one of these sets of laboratory tests, there are some particular considerations that should be pointed out. In the case of *electrolytes*, most of the decision levels are very close in value to the reference limits. This is not unexpected, in that these analytes are held very tightly for homeostatic purposes. Thus, even when a value differs only a little from the reference limit, we expect that physiologic aberrations will develop. Usually, the causes of such abnormalities relate to an imbalance in the regulation of input and output, perhaps due to a lack of control by one or more of the regulators. There are certain abnormalities in electrolyte values for which a very rapid decision must be made. In such cases, the decision levels could also be termed panic values. An extremely elevated plasma potassium and a very depressed serum calcium are two examples of panic values.

The second set of analytes consists of *metabolites.* With the exception of serum glucose, abnormalities in the metabolites do not usually demand rapid action. However, such abnormalities might signal the presence of an underlying disorder. Consequently, most of the action items in this category suggest additional diagnostic tests to exclude or confirm the clinical suspicion.

The third category consists of *proteins and enzymes.* Enzyme values differ dramatically, depending upon the laboratory method used. For example, some laboratories perform the enzyme test at 37°C, whereas others assay at 30°C. Going from 30° to 37° in the assay mixture may cause an increase of approximately 60 percent in the activity value. In addition, the presence or absence of cofactors, the buffer used, as well as the pH of the assay mixture all affect enzymatic activity. Thus, the reference values presented here should be used only as guidelines. If the reference values in your institution deviate from them, you can use a constant factor to adjust the decision levels appropriately.

There is a very high degree of variation in most enzyme activity values among healthy subjects. That is to say, a particular healthy subject may have an alkaline phosphatase value of 20 ± 5 U/L most of his adult life, and another may have a value of 80 ± 10 U/L most of his adult life. The differences between the two may relate to certain inherited attributes and have nothing whatsoever to do with the presence or absence of disease. Because of this high degree of interindividual variation in health as well as the possibility of following a slightly abnormal high value in the absence of disease, I have opted to use a decision level approximately 50 percent above the upper reference limit for most of the enzyme values and to consider all values above that threshold as results for which action should be instituted.

The next category consists of *hormone tests.* In clinical practice, results of these tests are usually examined in conjunction with other information. Such information includes other endocrine tests as well as the history and physical examination. Each test in this category is used to determine whether additional testing should be done to confirm or to exclude a suspected diagnosis.

The fifth category of tests is that of the *hematology-related analytes.* They are divided into the cellular components and plasma factors of hemostasis. Since there is relatively great variation for white cell counts, it's imperative that the clinical setting be taken into account.

The category of *miscellaneous tests* consists of a series of measurements for which reference values may not always be readily available. Thus it is important to see if these reference values are indeed appropriate for whatever method is used in a particular laboratory and to make what adjustments are necessary.

The final category of measurements considered is that of *drug tests*. Here, rather than giving reference intervals, I present therapeutic intervals. The therapeutic interval represents the range of values within which it is expected that the drug will have a reasonable physiologic effect without undue concern for side effects. Obviously, there are overlaps both on the low end as well as the high end of the therapeutic interval.

Decision levels for the drug assays are dependent upon whether there is evidence of adequate response to therapy as well as evidence of possible toxic effects from it. When there is evidence of reasonable response to therapy, there may be no need to increase the dosage. On the other hand, lack of response to therapy suggests that the dosage should be increased until the serum value reaches the next decision level or until there is either evidence of therapeutic response or of side effects (drug toxicity). When side effects that are consistent with the known toxic sequelae of a particular drug are observed, the decision level to stop or to decrease the dosage is lower than when no such clinical symptomatology is present. The decision levels here must, therefore, relate directly to the observed clinical setting.

Some objections or exceptions may be raised to the reference intervals proposed here as well as the specific decision levels recommended. For example, when determining values to be used for pediatric patients, the reference intervals may differ somewhat. Furthermore, the method or procedure used in the laboratory may affect the values, the reference interval, and then the decision level. The decision levels presented here may also be dependent somewhat on the therapy available in your institution, the economic considerations involved, as well as access to additional diagnostic testing such as is possible with sophisticated X-ray equipment. In spite of these exceptions, the concept of decision levels should be applicable in most clinical settings.

# PART

## TWO

# Decision Levels for Commonly Ordered Laboratory Tests

# 1

# Electrolytes

# CALCIUM

## Reference (normal) interval

9.0–10.6 mg/dl
(2.25–2.65 mmol/L)

## Causes of increased values

- Hyperparathyroidism
- Myeloma
- Metastatic carcinoma
- Sarcoidosis
- Thiazide therapy
- Thyrotoxicosis

## Causes of decreased values

- Hypoparathyroidism
- Hypoalbuminemia
- Chronic renal disease
- Acute pancreatitis
- Vitamin D deficiency
  (rickets, osteomalacia)
- Sprue steatorrhea
- Malnutrition

## DECISION LEVELS    ACTIONS

| 7.0 mg/dl |
|---|

Values below this level are associated with tetany. Depending upon the concentration of serum albumin, therapeutic actions must be considered.

| 11.0 mg/dl |
|---|

With values above this level, consider diagnostic measures to evaluate the hypercalcemia. A likely candidate is hyperparathyroidism.

| 13.5 mg/dl |
|---|

Values above this level are associated with toxicity—in this case, hypercalcemic coma. Vigorous therapeutic measures are indicated.

# CHLORIDE

## Reference (normal) interval

98–109 mmol/L

## Causes of increased values

- Prolonged diarrhea
- Renal tubular disease
- Hyperparathyroidism
- Dehydration

## Causes of decreased values

- Prolonged vomiting
- Burns
- Salt-losing renal diseases
- Overhydration
- Thiazide therapy

## DECISION LEVELS          ACTIONS

| 90 mmol/L |
|---|

With values below this level, the various causes of hypochloremia must be considered.

| 112 mmol/L |
|---|

With values above this level, the various causes of hyperchloremia must be considered. Additional diagnostic tests include serum sodium, potassium, calcium, and blood hematocrit.

# CO$_2$ CONTENT (HCO$_3^-$ + H$_2$CO$_3$)

## Reference (normal) interval

23–30 mmol/L

## Causes of increased values

- Primary metabolic alkalosis, as from vomiting, gastric suction, diuretic therapy, hypokalemia
- Primary respiratory acidosis, as from chronic pulmonary disease, airway obstruction, respiratory center depression, pulmonary emphysema

## Causes of decreased values

- Primary metabolic acidosis, as from diabetic ketoacidosis, uremia, starvation, lactic acidosis, alcoholic ketosis, salicylate ingestion
- Primary respiratory alkalosis, as from CNS stimulation, salicylate ingestion, psychogenic hyperventilation, arterial hypoxemia

| 6.0 mmol/L | Values below this level are usually associated with severe metabolic acidosis, with the blood pH often being less than 7.1. This is a medical emergency, and appropriate therapeutic measures are required. |

| 20 mmol/L | With values below this level, various causes for the decreased value must be considered, based, at least partially, on the actual blood pH. |

| 33 mmol/L | With values above this level, various causes for the increased value must be considered, based, at least partially, on the actual blood pII. |

|  |  |

|  |  |

# MAGNESIUM

## Reference (normal) interval

**1.2–2.4 mEq/L**
**(0.6–1.2 mmol/L)**

## Causes of increased values

- Renal disease
- Magnesium sulfate injection

## Causes of decreased values

- Alcoholism
- Malnutrition
- Malabsorption
- Severe diarrhea

| 1.2 mEq/L | Values at this level and lower are associated with weakness, irritability, tetany, and convulsions. The presence of these signs along with a decreased serum magnesium requires appropriate therapeutic measures. |

| 2.0 mEq/L | A value at this level is within the expected reference interval, and if hypomagnesemia had been considered a cause of the patient's clinical problem, other causes should be evaluated. |

| 5.0 mEq/L | A value at this level or greater is above the upper reference limit. Therapeutic measures must be considered. In addition, the presence of renal insufficiency should be assessed. |

# PHOSPHORUS

## Reference (normal) interval

**2.5–5.0 mg/dl**
**(0.81–1.62 mmol/L)**
Phosphorus is measured as the inorganic moiety.

## Causes of increased values

- Renal insufficiency
- Hypoparathyroidism
- Childhood
- Excess vitamin D intake
- High calcium diet

## Causes of decreased values

- Hyperparathyroidism (primary)
- Vitamin D deficiency
- Malabsorption
- Administration of glucose (hyperalimentation)
- Hyperinsulinism
- Loss of phosphate in urine, as in Fanconi's syndrome
- Insulin treatment of diabetic ketoacidosis
- Rickets
- Sprue steatorrhea

## DECISION LEVELS          ACTIONS

| 1.5 mg/dl | Values at this level or lower may be associated with hemolytic anemia. With such values, consider various therapeutic measures. |

| 2.5 mg/dl | This value is the lower reference limit. Values below this level would support the diagnosis of hyperparathyroidism in a patient with hypercalcemia. |

| 5.0 mg/dl | This value is the upper reference limit. Begin to consider various causes of this increased value. The presence of renal insufficiency should be assessed. |

# POTASSIUM

## Reference (normal) interval

3.7–5.3 mmol/L

## Causes of increased values

- Renal glomerular disease
- Adrenocortical insufficiency
- Diabetic ketoacidosis
- Excessive intravenous potassium therapy
- Sepsis
- Panhypopituitarism
- In vitro hemolysis

## Causes of decreased values

- Renal tubular disease
- Hyperaldosteronism
- Malnutrition
- Treatment of diabetic ketoacidosis
- Hyperinsulinism
- Metabolic alkalosis
- Diuretic therapy
- Gastrointestinal loss

## DECISION LEVELS          ACTIONS

| 3.0 mmol/L | This is below the lower reference limit. Values below this level may be associated with weakness, digoxin toxicity, and/or cardiac arrhythmias. Consider appropriate therapeutic measures. |

| 5.8 mmol/L | This is above the upper reference limit. Consider further diagnostic measures. The presence of renal glomerular disease should be considered. In vitro hemolysis should be ruled out. |

| 7.5 mmol/L | Any value higher than this level may be associated with cardiac arrhythmias. Consider appropriate therapeutic measures. In vitro hemolysis should be ruled out. |

# SODIUM

### Reference (normal) interval

138–146 mmol/L

### Causes of increased values

- Dehydration
- Diabetes insipidus (loss of dilute urine)
- Loss of hypotonic gastrointestinal fluids
- Salt poisoning
- Peritoneal dialysis with hypertonic glucose solution
- Selective depression of sense of thirst
- Skin losses, burns, sweating
- Hyperaldosteronism
- CNS disorders, as with meningitis, stroke, trauma, neurosurgical procedures

### Causes of decreased values

- Dilutional hyponatremia, as with cirrhosis, congestive heart failure, water overload
- Depletional hyponatremia, as with salt-losing nephritis, tubular lesions, diuretic therapy, adrenal insufficiency, gastrointestinal loss, sweating
- Syndrome of inappropriate ADH secretion
- Delusional hyponatremia, as with hyperlipidemia or greatly increased serum protein.

| 115 mmol/L |
|---|

At this value or lower, there may be mental confusion, fatigue, headache, nausea, vomiting, and anorexia. At a value of 110 mmol/L, the patient is vulnerable to convulsions, semicoma, or coma. Given a value of 115 mmol/L, it's imperative to determine the level of hydration and to treat the patient accordingly.

| 135 mmol/L |
|---|

This value is below the lower reference limit. The various causes of hyponatremia must be considered. Additional diagnostic tests to be ordered include serum osmolality, potassium, and urine studies.

| 150 mmol/L |
|---|

This value is above the upper reference limit. The various causes of the hypernatremia must be considered.

| |
|---|

# 2

# Metabolites

# BILIRUBIN

## Reference (normal) interval

0.1–1.2 mg/dl
(1.7–20.5 μmol/L)

## Causes of increased values    Causes of decreased values

- Liver insufficiency
- Extrahepatic obstruction
- Hemolysis
- In neonate, due to a variety
  of causes including
  neonatal physiological
  hyperbilirubinemia
- Gilbert's disease

## DECISION LEVELS          ACTIONS

| 1.4 mg/dl | Values at this level are above the reference interval. Consider various causes of hyperbilirubinemia. Serum AST (SGOT), prothrombin time, and serum ALP can help to rule in or rule out liver disease. |

| 2.5 mg/dl | Values above this level are associated with jaundice. In any patient who appears jaundiced, a serum bilirubin below this level suggests an alternative cause for the condition. |

| 20 mg/dl | In infants, a serum bilirubin above this level is often associated with brain damage (kernicterus). Therapeutic maneuvers, e.g., blood transfusions, should be considered, based on additional clinical and/or laboratory information. |

# CHOLESTEROL

## Reference (normal) interval

150–250 mg/dl
(3.9–6.5 mmol/L)

## Causes of increased values

- Familial (hereditary) hypercholesterolemia
- Biliary obstruction
- Nephrotic syndrome
- Hypothyroidism
- Pregnancy

## Causes of decreased values

- Severe liver insufficiency
- Malnutrition
- Hyperthyroidism
- Chronic anemia
- Waldenström's macroglobulinemia
- Thyroiditis

## DECISION LEVELS    ACTIONS

| 90 mg/dl |
|---|

Values below this level are often associated with severe liver insufficiency. With such values, appropriate diagnostic and therapeutic measures must be considered. If there is known liver disease, a finding below this level may indicate a very bad prognosis.

| 250 mg/dl |
|---|

This is the upper reference limit for a young adult male. Values above this level may represent a risk factor for atherosclerotic cardiovascular disease. Appropriate advice to the patient should be given.

| 400 mg/dl |
|---|

Values above this level represent very serious prognostic implications regarding atherosclerotic cardiovascular disease. Therapeutic measures, e.g., diet, drugs, surgery, must be considered.

# CREATININE

## Reference (normal) interval

**0.7–1.5 mg/dl (adults)**
**(62–133 $\mu$mol/L)**

## Causes of increased values

- Impaired renal function (serum creatinine is a more specific indicator of renal disease than is serum urea)

## Causes of decreased values

- Rare and not clinically significant

**0.6 mg/dl**

In infants, a value above this level is considered above the age-specific expected reference interval, and renal insufficiency must be considered. Further measurements of renal function should be evaluated.

**1.6 mg/dl**

Values at this level or greater are above the expected adult reference interval. Consider ordering further measurements of renal function, e.g., creatinine clearance test.

**6.0 mg/dl**

Values above this level are almost invariably associated with severe renal impairment. The prognostic significance of the value must be assessed and the appropriate therapeutic regimen initiated.

# GLUCOSE

## Reference (normal) interval

60–95 mg/dl
(3.33–5.28 mmol/L)

## Causes of increased values

- Diabetes mellitus
    Maturity-onset (adult)
    Growth-onset (juvenile)
- Pancreatitis
- Endocrine disorders, as in acromegaly, Cushing's syndrome, thyrotoxicosis, pheochromocytoma, hyperaldosteronism
- Drugs such as steroids, thiazides, oral contraceptives
- Chronic renal failure
- Stress
- IV glucose infusion
- Postprandial testing

## Causes of decreased values

- Insulinoma
- Adrenocortical insufficiency
- Hypopituitarism
- Extrapancreatic neoplasms
- Massive liver disease
- Ethanol ingestion
- Drug ingestion, as with sulfonylurea, salicylates, phenformin, insulin
- Reactive hypoglycemia
    Functional hypoglycemia
    Prediabetic hypoglycemia
    Alimentary hypoglycemia
- Glycogen storage disease of the newborn (Type I)

## DECISION LEVELS        ACTIONS

| 45 mg/dl | A value at this level or less after a 12-hour fast is considered consistent with a diagnosis of hypoglycemia. Appropriate therapeutic measures should be considered. Such values are associated with anxiety, shakiness, sweating, trembling, and weakness. If the reaction occurs slowly, headache, irritability, and lethargy predominate. Appropriate diagnostic measures should be considered to identify the etiology. |

| 120 mg/dl | A value at this level or greater in a plasma specimen obtained from a fasting patient has been used as a criterion to suggest the diagnosis of diabetes. A glucose tolerance test may be indicated. |

| 180 mg/dl | A value at this level or greater in a plasma specimen obtained one hour after a meal is highly indicative of diabetes. However, investigators differ in the criteria (cutoff values) used to make the diagnosis of diabetes. |

# IRON

## Reference (normal) interval

50–165 μg/dl
(9.0–29.5 μmol/L)

## Causes of increased values

- Hemochromatosis
- Hemosiderosis of excessive iron intake
- Decreased formation of RBCs, as with thalassemia, pyridoxine-deficiency anemia
- Hemolytic anemias
- Acute liver damage
- Iron ingestion

## Causes of decreased values

- Iron-deficiency anemia (hypochromic, microcytic)
- Late pregnancy
- Chronic infections
- Menstruation
- Nephrosis
- Kwashiorkor

| DECISION LEVELS | ACTIONS |
|---|---|

| 50 μg/dl | Values at this level or below are associated with iron-deficiency anemia. The presence of microcytic, hypochromic RBCs and an elevation of total iron-binding capacity (TIBC) must be documented. A low serum ferritin is helpful when the TIBC value is equivocal. |
|---|---|
| 220 μg/dl | Values at this level or above are associated with various pathologies. Appropriate diagnostic and therapeutic measures should be considered. |
| 400 μg/dl | A value at this level or above in a patient who has ingested an overdose of iron is a grave prognostic sign. Appropriate therapeutic measures should be considered. |

# UREA NITROGEN (BUN)

## Reference (normal) interval

8–26 mg/dl
(2.9–9.3 mmol/L)

## Causes of increased values

- Impaired renal function
- Prerenal azotemia, as with congestive heart failure, shock
- Postrenal azotemia
- Gastrointestinal bleeding
- High-protein diet
- Drugs (corticosteroids, tetracycline)

## Causes of decreased values

- Pregnancy (third trimester)
- Severe liver insufficiency
- Overhydration
- Malnutrition, especially decreased protein intake
- Lipoid nephrosis

| DECISION LEVELS | ACTIONS |
| --- | --- |

| 6 mg/dl | Values below this level are frequently associated with states of overhydration or hepatic insufficiency. |
| --- | --- |

| 26 mg/dl | This value is the upper reference limit. With higher values, the various causes of an increased serum urea nitrogen must be considered. A serum creatinine would be helpful in assessing renal function. |
| --- | --- |

| 50 mg/dl | Values above this level are very often associated with severe renal impairment. Appropriate diagnostic and/or therapeutic alternatives must be chosen. Renal disease, if present, should be characterized. |
| --- | --- |

# URIC ACID (URATE)

## Reference (normal) interval

2.5–7.0 mg/dl
(0.15–0.41 mmol/L)

## Causes of increased values

- Gout
- Renal failure
- Ketoacidosis
- Lactate excess, as after ethanol ingestion
- Diuretic therapy
- Lesch-Nyhan syndrome
- Chronic lead nephropathy
- Polycystic kidneys
- Leukemia, lymphoma, polycythemia
- Diet (high-protein, high-nucleoprotein)
- Antiuricosuric drugs such as diuretics

## Causes of decreased values

- Administration of ACTH
- Administration of uricosuric drugs (high doses of salicylates, probenecid, cortisone, allo-purinol, coumarin)
- Renal tubular defects (Fanconi's syndrome, Wilson's disease)

| 2.0 mg/dl |
|---|

This value is below the lower reference limit. With it or any lower value, consider various diagnostic measures to appropriately classify the patient.

| 8.0 mg/dl |
|---|

This value is above the upper reference limit. With it or any higher value, consider various diagnostic measures to appropriately classify the patient.

| 10.7 mg/dl |
|---|

With values at this level or above, there is an increased risk to form renal calculi or joint tophi. Appropriate therapeutic measures should be considered.

# 3

# Proteins and Enzymes

# ALANINE AMINOTRANSFERASE (ALT, SGPT)

## Reference (normal) interval

5–40 U/L at 37°C

## Causes of increased values

- Viral hepatitis
- Toxic hepatitis
- Shock liver
- Infectious mononucleosis
- Alcoholic hepatitis
- Polymyositis

## Causes of decreased values

- End stage liver disease
- Renal hemodialysis
- Renal insufficiency

## DECISION LEVELS    ACTIONS

| 20 U/L |
|--------|

A value at this level is within the reference interval and would rule out a number of entities associated with increased ALT. Other diagnoses should be considered. Such values within the normal interval can be compared with past and/or future values when the patient is used as his own control.

| 60 U/L |
|--------|

With values at this level or above, various causes for the elevated result must be considered.

| 300 U/L |
|---------|

A value above this level is most often consistent with acute hepatocellular injury, e.g., viral hepatitis, toxic hepatitis, shock liver. Most other causes of increased ALT, e.g., alcoholic hepatitis, are associated with lower values.

## ALBUMIN

### Reference (normal) interval

3.5–5.0 g/dl
(35–50 g/L)

### Causes of increased values

- Dehydration

### Causes of decreased values

- Renal disease—nephrotic syndrome with protein loss in urine
- Liver insufficiency with decreased albumin synthesis
- Severe malnutrition
- Acute inflammation
- Chronic inflammation
- Malignancy
- Pregnancy
- Burns

## DECISION LEVELS · ACTIONS

| 2.0 g/dl | A value below this level is a serious prognostic finding in a patient with liver disease. Measure for urinary protein to confirm excessive protein loss. |

| 3.5 g/dl | With values below this lower reference limit, various causes of decreased serum albumin must be considered. |

| 5.2 g/dl | With values above this level, the possibility of dehydration must be considered. An increased hematocrit would be consistent with that diagnosis. |

# ALKALINE PHOSPHATASE (ALP)

## Reference (normal) interval

35–120 U/L at 37°C (adults)
50–400 U/L at 37°C (children)

## Causes of increased values

- Intrahepatic cholestasis, as with carcinoma infiltrating into the liver, leukemia, tuberculosis, sarcoidosis, amyloidosis, fibrosis (cirrhosis)
- Extrahepatic cholestasis, as with bile duct stone, neoplasm, biliary atresia
- Osteoblastic disease such as metastatic bone disease, secondary hyperparathyroidism
- Alkaline phosphatase-producing tumor
- Pregnancy

## Causes of decreased values

- Hypophosphatemia (relatively rare)

| 50 U/L |
|---|

A value at this level is within the reference interval and would rule out a number of entities associated with increased ALP. Other diagnoses should be considered. Such values within the normal interval can be compared with past and/or future values when the patient is used as his own control.

| 150 U/L |
|---|

A value at this level or greater is above the adult reference interval. Various causes of the increased ALP must be considered. Additional diagnostic tests may be needed to classify the patient into the appropriate clinical group. A serum GGT value could be helpful in the workup of the patient.

| 400 U/L |
|---|

A value greater than this level is above the pediatric reference interval. Various causes of the increased ALP must be considered. Additional diagnostic tests may be needed to classify the patient into the appropriate clinical group.

|  |
|---|

# AMYLASE

## Reference (normal) interval

60–180 Somogyi units
(110–330 U/L)

## Causes of increased values

- Pancreatitis
- Perforated or penetrating peptic ulcer
- Acute ethanol ingestion
- Salivary gland disease (mumps, inflammation)
- Obstruction of pancreatic duct
- Severe renal disease
- Macroamylasemia
- Stone in the common bile duct
- Spasm of the common bile duct

## Causes of decreased values

- Extensive destruction of the pancreas
- Marked hepatic insufficiency

## DECISION LEVELS        ACTIONS

| 50 Somogyi units |
|---|

A value at this level or below in a patient with liver disease is a very serious prognostic finding. Appropriate therapeutic measures should be considered, if the diagnosis of liver disease has been confirmed.

| 120 Somogyi units |
|---|

This value is within the expected reference interval. Values below it should rule out a diagnosis of acute pancreatitis in most cases. Other diagnostic entities should be considered if appropriate.

| 200 Somogyi units |
|---|

A value at this level or greater is above the upper reference interval. The diagnosis of acute pancreatitis can be entertained if supported by appropriate clinical and laboratory data.

# ASPARTATE AMINOTRANSFERASE (AST, SGOT)

## Reference (normal) interval

8–40 U/L at 37°C

## Causes of increased values

- Hepatocellular destruction, as in viral hepatitis, toxic hepatitis, shock liver, alcoholic hepatitis
- Myocardial infarction
- In vivo hemolysis
- Musculoskeletal disease
- Pulmonary infarction
- Posthepatic obstructive biliary tract disease

## Causes of decreased values

- End stage liver disease
- Chronic hemodialysis
- Pregnancy

## DECISION LEVELS        ACTIONS

| 20 U/L |
|---|

A value near this level is within the reference interval and would rule out a number of entities associated with increased AST. Other diagnoses should be considered. Such values within the normal interval can be compared with past and/or future values when the patient is used as his own control.

| 60 U/L |
|---|

A value at this level or greater is above the upper reference limit for AST. Various causes for the elevated result must be considered. Helpful diagnostic tests include ALT, ALP, bilirubin, and CK.

| 300 U/L |
|---|

A value above this level is most often consistent with acute hepatocellular injury, e.g., viral hepatitis, toxic hepatitis. Most other causes of increased AST, e.g., alcoholic hepatitis, myocardial infarction, progressive muscular dystrophy, are associated with lower values.

# CARCINOEMBRYONIC ANTIGEN (CEA)

## Reference (normal) interval

<2.5 ng/ml
(<2.5 µg/L)

CEA value is very assay-dependent.

## Causes of increased values

- Malignancy
- Liver disease
    Acute hepatitis
    Alcoholic cirrhosis
    Extrahepatic biliary
    obstruction
- Acute pancreatitis
- Regional enteritis
- Ulcerative colitis
- Pulmonary emphysema
- Chronic bronchitis
- Bacterial pneumonia
- Pulmonary tuberculosis
- Smoking

## Causes of decreased values

- Not applicable

## DECISION LEVELS ACTIONS

| 2.5 ng/ml | In a patient in whom a CEA-producing neoplasm has been documented, a value below this level would be consistent with a good prognosis. It is recommended to follow such patients with sequential monitoring. |

| 10.0 ng/ml | In the absence of nonneoplastic causes of increased CEA values, a value at this level or greater would suggest a possible malignancy. A workup for a gastrointestinal neoplasm would be in order. |

| 20.0 ng/ml | In the absence of severe hepatic disease, a CEA value above this level in a patient known to have malignancy would strongly suggest recurrence. Appropriate therapeutic intervention would be indicated. |

# CREATINE KINASE (CK)

## Reference (normal) interval

10–180 U/L at 37°C

## Causes of increased values

- Myocardial infarction
- Progressive muscular dystrophy
- Dermatomyositis
- Rhabdomyolysis due to drug ingestion, hyperosmolality, autoimmune disease, etc.
- Delirium tremens
- Convulsions (status epilepticus)
- Crush syndrome
- Hypothyroidism
- Surgery
- Severe exercise
- Intramuscular injection

## Causes of decreased values

- Physical inactivity
- Decreased muscle mass

## DECISION LEVELS    ACTIONS

100 U/L

A value at this level or below is within the reference interval and would rule out a number of entities associated with increased CK. Other diagnoses should be considered. Such values within the normal interval can be compared with past and/or future values when the patient is used as his own control.

240 U/L

A value above this level is consistent with what can be expected 1–2 days after acute myocardial infarction. Appropriate diagnostic procedures, e.g., CK isoenzyme determinations, should be considered.

1800 U/L

A value above this level is most often seen in pathological entities other than uncomplicated acute myocardial infarction, e.g., rhabdomyolysis, delirium tremens, status epilepticus. Consider diagnostic measures to support or reject the possible diagnostic classes.

# GLUTAMYL TRANSFERASE (GGT)

## Reference (normal) interval

5–40 U/L at 37°C

## Causes of increased values

- Hepatobiliary disease
- History of ethanol ingestion
- History of drug ingestion, as with phenytoin, phenobarbital

## Causes of decreased values

- Rare and not clinically significant

## DECISION LEVELS          ACTIONS

20 U/L

A value at this level is within the reference interval and would rule out a number of entities associated with increased GGT. Other diagnoses should be considered. Such values within the normal interval can be compared with past and/or future values when the patient is used as his own control.

50 U/L

With values above this level, various causes of the increased GGT must be considered. Values between this level and the next one in the presence of a normal ALP may signify prior ethanol and/or drug ingestion.

150 U/L

A value above this level is most often associated with hepatobiliary disease. Various diagnostic and therapeutic measures should be considered.

# LACTATE DEHYDROGENASE (LDH)

## Reference (normal) interval

**60–220 U/L at 37°C**
lactate ⟶ pyruvate

## Causes of increased values

- Hemolytic disease such as megaloblastic anemia, sickle cell anemia
- Myocardial infarction
- Malignancy, e.g., leukemia, lymphoma, metastatic carcinoma
- Pulmonary infarction
- Infectious mononucleosis
- Progressive muscular dystrophy
- Delirium tremens
- Trauma
- Shock liver
- Hepatic disorders

## Causes of decreased values

- Rare and not clinically significant

## DECISION LEVELS    ACTIONS

| 150 U/L |
|---|

A value at this level or lower is within the reference interval and would rule out a number of entities associated with increased LDH. Other diagnoses should be considered. Such values within the normal interval can be compared with past and/or future values when the patient is used as his own control.

| 300 U/L |
|---|

With values above this level, consider various causes of increased LDH. Appropriate diagnostic tests should be ordered.

| 500 U/L |
|---|

Values above this level are most often seen in megaloblastic anemia, acute leukemia, chronic granulocytic leukemia, metastatic carcinoma, trauma, and shock liver. Certain tests should be considered to discover the correct diagnosis.

# TOTAL PROTEIN

## Reference (normal) interval

6.0–8.0 g/dl
(60–80 g/L)

## Causes of increased values

- Dehydration
- Chronic inflammation
- Myeloma (IgG, IgA)
- Sarcoidosis

## Causes of decreased values

- Overhydration
- Hepatic insufficiency
- Malnutrition
- Myeloma (light chain)
- Agammaglobulinemia
- Malignancy
- Nephrotic syndrome
- Protein-losing enteropathy

## DECISION LEVELS        ACTIONS

4.5 g/dl

A value below this level may be associated with peripheral edema. Appropriate therapeutic measures should be considered. Moreover, tests of urine protein excretion, hepatic function, and fluid balance may be appropriate.

6.0 g/dl

With a value at this lower reference limit or below, various causes for the depressed result must be considered. Appropriate diagnostic measures should be chosen, as noted above.

8.0 g/dl

A value greater than this level is above the upper reference limit. Various causes for the elevated result must be considered. Appropriate diagnostic measures, including a serum protein electrophoresis, should be ordered.

# 4

# Hormones

# CORTISOL (FREE) IN URINE

## Reference (normal) interval

**20–90 μg/24 hours**
**(55–248 nmol/24 hours)**

## Causes of increased values

- Cushing's syndrome
- Exogenous steroids
- Starvation
- Hydration in the form of water loading
- Emotional or physical stress

## Causes of decreased values

- Adrenocortical insufficiency (Addison's disease)
- Renal disease
- Incomplete collection

50 $\mu$g/24 hours

Values below this level run counter to the hypothesis that the patient suffers from Cushing's syndrome. Other diagnoses should be considered. Note: Undetected free cortisol in urine does not preclude normal adrenal function.

100 $\mu$g/24 hours

Values greater than this level are very suggestive of Cushing's syndrome. A low-dose (1 mg) dexamethasone test can confirm the diagnosis. (For additional information, see Cortisol in Plasma, pages 80–81.)

# FOLLICLE-STIMULATING HORMONE (FSH)

## Reference (normal) interval

Prepubertal males
1–3 mIU/ml

Prepubertal females
1–3 mIU/ml

Adult males
2–15 mIU/ml

Adult females
| Follicular phase | 3–15 mIU/ml |
| Ovulatory spike | 10–50 mIU/ml |
| Luteal phase | 3–15 mIU/ml |
| Postmenopause | 30–200 mIU/ml |

## Causes of increased values

Primary testicular failure
- Adult seminiferous tubular failure
- Myotonic dystrophy
- Congenital anorchia and agonadism
- Sertoli's cells only

Ovarian failure
- Premature menopause

Chromosomal disorders
*In males*
- Klinefelter's syndrome
- XYY
- Mixed gonadal dysgenesis
- Male Turner's syndrome
- True hermaphroditism
*In females*
- Turner's syndrome
- Pure gonadal dysgenesis
- Mixed gonadal dysgenesis
- True hermaphroditism

Other causes
- Pseudohermaphroditism (testicular feminization)
- Alcoholism

## Causes of decreased values

- Hypopituitarism
- Kallmann's syndrome
- Delayed puberty
- Postpregnancy
- Oral contraceptive use
- Hypothalamic lesions
- Anorexia nervosa
- Emotional or physical stress
- Hemochromatosis
- Prolactinoma
- Prader-Willi syndrome

## DECISION LEVELS          ACTIONS

| 1 mIU/ml |
|---|

Values below this level would suggest ordering a serum testosterone or estradiol to confirm a hypogonadotropic-hypogonadal state. Subsequent studies might include serum prolactin, growth hormone stimulation test, and serum thyroxine assays as well as GRH stimulation tests.

| 35 mIU/ml in adult males |
|---|

Values above this level in a young adult male may represent primary testicular failure. A serum testosterone should be ordered to confirm this. The reference interval for serum testosterone in adult men is 300–1100 ng/dl.

| 60 mIU/ml in adult females |
|---|

Values above this level in an adult female (excluding ovulatory spike) may represent primary ovarian failure. A serum estradiol should be ordered to confirm this.

# 17-HYDROXYCORTICOSTEROIDS IN URINE

## Reference (normal) interval

3–10 mg/24 hours

## Causes of increased values

- Cushing's syndrome
- Severe stress
- Numerous drug interferences
- Pregnancy (last trimester)
- Hyperthyroidism

## Causes of decreased values

- Adrenocortical insufficiency
- Anterior pituitary hypofunction
- Hypothyroidism

## DECISION LEVELS      ACTIONS

| 3 mg/24 hours |
|---|

A value below this level after a low-dose (1 mg) dexamethasone suppression test rules out Cushing's syndrome in the patient.

| 15 mg/24 hours in females |
|---|

Values above this level in a female are consistent with Cushing's syndrome. Due to the nonspecificity of this test, a urinary free cortisol test is recommended to support the diagnosis of Cushing's syndrome.

| 20 mg/24 hours in males |
|---|

Values above this level in a male are consistent with Cushing's syndrome. Due to the nonspecificity of this test, a urinary free cortisol test is recommended to support the diagnosis of Cushing's syndrome.

# 17-KETOSTEROIDS IN URINE

## Reference (normal) interval

5–15 mg/24 hours (adult females)
8–20 mg/24 hours (adult males)

0.1–3.0 mg/24 hours (prepubertal children)

## Causes of increased values

- Ovarian tumors
    Arrhenoblastoma
    Luteal cell tumor
- Interstitial (Leydig) cell tumor of testes
- Adrenocortical excess, as in carcinoma, adenoma, hyperplasia
- Pregnancy (last trimester)
- Severe stress
- Testosterone administration
- ACTH administration
- Virilization syndrome
- Stein-Leventhal syndrome
- Adrenogenital syndrome
- Numerous drug interferences

## Causes of decreased values

- Adrenocortical insufficiency
- Testicular hypofunction
    Primary hypogonadism
    Secondary hypogonadism
- Nephrotic syndrome
- Anterior pituitary hypofunction
- Female hypogonadism
- Prepubertal children

## DECISION LEVELS      ACTIONS

| 20 mg/24 hours |
|---|

Values in excess of this level in adult females suggest adrenal or ovarian origin for hirsutism. A low-dose (1 mg) dexamethasone suppression test of adrenal output, which can indicate the cause, is advisable. DHEAS is a better indicator of adrenal androgen output.

| 25 mg/24 hours |
|---|

Values above this level in a newborn male with accentuation of genitalia or a female with masculinization of the genitalia suggest the adrenogenital syndrome. A urinary pregnanetriol should be ordered. If it is elevated, cortisol-like therapy should be instituted.

| 40 mg/24 hours |
|---|

Values above this level suggest Cushing's syndrome. Further tests include AM and PM plasma cortisol, urinary free cortisol, and low-dose (1 mg) dexamethasone suppression test (in that order).

# LUTEINIZING HORMONE (LH)

## Reference (normal) interval

Prepubertal males
2–6 mIUL/ml

Prepubertal females
2–6 mIU/ml

Adult males
5–25 mIU/ml

Adult females
Follicular phase   5–30 mIU/ml
Ovulatory spike   50–150 mIU/ml
Luteal phase   5–40 mIU/ml
Postmenopause   30–200 mIU/ml

## Causes of increased values

Primary testicular failure
- Congenital anorchia and agonadism
- Adult Leydig-cell failure

Ovarian failure
- Premature menopause

Chromosomal disorders
*In males*
- Klinefelter's syndrome
- XYY
- Mixed gonadal dysgenesis
- Male Turner's syndrome
- True hermaphroditism
*In females*
- Turner's syndrome
- Pure gonadal dysgenesis
- Mixed gonadal dysgenesis
- True hermaphroditism

Other causes
- Pseudohermaphroditism (testicular feminization)
- Polycystic ovaries
- Alcoholism
- Ectopic hormone syndromes, as in hepatoma, testicular tumor, lung cancer

## Causes of decreased values

- Hypopituitarism
- Kallmann's syndrome
- Delayed puberty
- Postpregnancy
- Oral contraceptive use
- Hypothalamic lesions
- Anorexia nervosa
- Emotional or physical stress
- Fertile eunuch syndrome
- Hemochromatosis

## DECISION LEVELS    ACTIONS

| 1 mIU/ml |
|---|

Values below this level would suggest ordering a serum testosterone or estradiol to confirm a hypogonadotropic-hypogonadal state. Subsequent studies might include serum prolactin, growth hormone stimulation test, and serum thyroxine assays, as well as GRH stimulation test.

| 50 mIU/ml in adult males |
|---|

Values above this level in a young male adult may represent primary testicular failure. A serum testosterone should be ordered to confirm this. The reference interval for serum testosterone in adult men is 300–1100 ng/dl.

| 100 mIU/ml in adult females |
|---|

Values above this level in an adult female (excluding ovulatory spike) may represent primary ovarian failure. A serum estradiol should be ordered to confirm this. The diagnosis of polycystic ovaries would be supported by an elevated serum testosterone or an elevated urinary 17-ketosteroids value.

# METANEPHRINE IN URINE

## Reference (normal) interval

<1.3 mg/24 hours

## Causes of increased values   Causes of decreased values

- Neuroblastoma
- Pheochromocytoma
- Severe stress
    Hemorrhagic shock
    Sepsis
    Widespread metastatic
      disease
- Monoamine oxidase inhibitors

| 1.3 mg/24 hours | Values below this level in combination with normal VMA and normal urinary free catecholamines exclude the diagnosis of pheochromocytoma in 95% of cases. Values above this level in conjunction with other supporting evidence would suggest arteriography to confirm and to localize the tumor. |

| 2.5 mg/24 hours | Values above this level are diagnostic—confirmatory—of a catecholamine-producing tumor (pheochromocytoma, neuroblastoma, ganglioneuroma, or ganglioblastoma), provided there is no possibility of interference due to drugs and/or diet. The tumor should be localized by angiography and it should be excised surgically. |

# PROLACTIN

## Reference (normal) interval

1–20 ng/ml (males)
(1–20 μg/L)

1–25 ng/ml (females)
(1–25 μg/L)

## Causes of increased values

Physiologic
•Newborn
•Pregnancy
•Postpartum
•Stress
•Exercise
•Sleep
•Nipple stimulation
Drugs
•Phenothiazines
•Estrogens
•Reserpine
•Alpha-methyldopa
•Haloperidol
•Benzamides
•Pimozide
•Thyrotropin releasing hormone
  (TRH)
•Meprobamate
•Tricyclic antidepressants
Pathologic
•Prolactin-secreting tumors
•Acromegaly
•Hypothalamic disorders
•Pituitary stalk section
•Hypothyroidism
•Renal failure
•Ectopic production by malignant
  tumors

## Causes of decreased values

• Pituitary necrosis
• Pituitary infarction

## DECISION LEVELS ACTIONS

| 30 ng/ml |
| --- |

Values above this level may be associated with various physiological and pharmacological causes as well as related to serious pathology. If patient is on drug that causes an increase in prolactin, temporary cessation of drug and repeat testing may be advisable.

| 100 ng/ml |
| --- |

Values above this level are generally associated with pituitary tumors, especially in combination with galactorrhea. Aggressive additional diagnostic testing should be pursued to confirm that diagnosis.

| 300 ng/ml |
| --- |

A value above this level in association with galactorrhea confirms the diagnosis of pituitary tumor in virtually 100% of cases. Appropriate therapy should be instituted.

# THYROXINE (T$_4$)

## Reference (normal) interval

**5.5–12.5 $\mu$g/dl (adults)**
**(72 to 163 nmol/L)**

**7.8–16.0 $\mu$g/dl (newborns)**
**(101 to 208 nmol/L)**

## Causes of increased values

With normal free T$_4$ index
(elevated TBG)
• Pregnancy
• Oral contraceptive use
• Estrogen therapy
Hyperthyroidism
• Diffuse toxic goiter (Graves'
  disease)
• Toxic goiter
• Exogenous thyroid hormone
  excess
• Tumors, i.e., thyroxine
  producing, TSH-like substance
  producing

## Causes of decreased values

With normal free T$_4$ index
(decreased TBG)
• Malnutrition
• Nephrotic syndrome
• Severe liver disease
• Phenytoin, salicylates
• Androgens, anabolic steroids
Congenital hypothyroidism
• Primary
• Secondary
Acquired hypothyroidism
• Primary— ↑TSH
• Secondary— ↓TSH, and not
  responsive to TRF
• Tertiary— ↓TSH, but responsive
  to TRF

| 5 $\mu$g/dl in nonpregnant adults | Values below this level in an adult suspected of being hypothyroid would suggest ordering a free T$_4$ index. A confirmatory elevated TSH value should initiate appropriate thyroxine-replacement therapy. |

| 7 $\mu$g/dl on third day of life | Values below this level in a newborn screened for hypothyroidism suggest ordering a TSH to substantiate the diagnosis. With elevated TSH values, thyroid therapy should be instituted. |

| 10 $\mu$g/dl in nonpregnant adults | Values above this level in an adult suspected of being hyperthyroid would suggest ordering a free T$_4$ index. If free T$_4$ is elevated, appropriate therapy should be given. If free T$_4$ is not elevated, a T$_3$ test may be ordered to rule out T$_3$ thyrotoxicosis. |

| 14 $\mu$g/dl in nonpregnant adults | In the absence of pregnancy, estrogen therapy, or taking of oral contraceptives, values above this level are almost always consistent with hyperthyroidism. If clinical symptomatology supports the diagnosis, therapy can begin immediately. |

# VANILLYLMANDELIC ACID (VMA) IN URINE

## Reference (normal) interval

<6.8 mg/24 hours

## Causes of increased values

- Neuroblastoma
- Pheochromocytoma
- Dietary intake of vanilla, bananas, coffee, tea, chocolate
- Exercise stress

Drugs
  *Physiologic effect*
- Epinephrine
- Lithium carbonate
- Nitroglycerin
  *Chemical interference (method-dependent)*
- Anileridine
- Caffeine
- Methenamine mandelate
- Methocarbamol
- Salicylates

## Causes of decreased values

Drugs
- Methyldopa
- Monoamine oxidase inhibitors
- Clofibrate
- Guanethidine analogs
- Imipramine

| DECISION LEVELS | ACTIONS |
| --- | --- |

| 6.8 mg/24 hours | Values below this level in combination with normal urinary metanephrine and normal urinary free catecholamines exclude the diagnosis of pheochromocytoma in 95% of cases. Values above this level in conjunction with other supporting evidence would suggest arteriography to confirm and to localize the tumor. |
| --- | --- |
| 13 mg/24 hours | Values above this level are diagnostic—confirmatory—of a catecholamine-producing tumor (pheochromocytoma, neuroblastoma, ganglioneuroma, or ganglioblastoma), provided there is no possibility of interference due to drugs and/or diet. The tumor should be localized by angiography and it should be excised surgically. |

# 5

# Hematology-Related Tests

# ANTITHROMBIN-III (AT-III)

## Reference (normal) interval

80–120% of normal human pooled plasma (NHPP)

| Causes of increased values | Causes of decreased values |
| --- | --- |
| | • Thrombosis |
| | • Hypercoagulable state |
| | • Disseminated intravascular coagulation (DIC) |
| | • Hereditary deficiency |
| | • Use of oral contraceptives |
| | • Liver disease |
| | • Nephrotic syndrome |
| | • Surgery/trauma |
| | • Heparin therapy |
| | • Asparaginase therapy |

## DECISION LEVELS  ACTIONS

50% of NHPP

Values below this level are often associated with spontaneous thrombosis. When heparinizing such patients, additional dosage may be necessary. Heparin therapy should be monitored via PTT or activated clotting time.

75% of NHPP

Values below this level suggest ordering additional tests, e.g., PT, platelet count, and fibrinogen to support the diagnosis of DIC.

# BLEEDING TIME

### Reference (normal) interval

0–6 minutes (Simplate®)

### Causes of shortened values    ### Causes of prolonged values

- Thrombocytopenia
- Platelet dysfunction
- Von Willebrand's disease
- Salicylate ingestion
- Ingestion of other anti-inflammatory drugs, e.g., indomethacin, ibuprofen, phenylbutazone

## DECISION LEVELS    ACTIONS

| 6 minutes |
|---|

Values above this level suggest either thrombocytopenia, platelet dysfunction, or von Willebrand's disease. Additional tests of platelet count, APTT, and, if necessary, platelet aggregation should be ordered. Prolonged APTT is associated with von Willebrand's disease. Platelet counts of 50,000/$\mu$l or less are usually associated with prolonged bleeding time.

| 8 minutes |
|---|

If patient is to undergo major surgery and the bleeding time is higher than this level, then correctional therapy before and immediately after surgery will be required.

| 15 minutes |
|---|

A value in excess of this level is associated with serious, uncontrollable hemorrhage in 73% of patients when platelets are less than 10,000/$\mu$l. Therapy should be administered in the form of platelets, if platelet insufficiency is indicated as the cause of the prolonged bleeding time.

# FIBRINOGEN IN PLASMA

## Reference (normal) interval

200–400 mg/dl
(2–4 g/L)

## Causes of increased values

- Acute infection
- Collagen diseases, e.g., rheumatoid arthritis
- Nephrosis
- Hepatitis without severe liver damage
- Radiation therapy
- Burns
- Surgery (after 5–10 days)
- Pyrexia (after 1–4 days)
- Myocardial infarction
- Pregnancy

## Causes of decreased values

- Congenital afibrinogenemia, hypofibrinogenemia, or dysfibrinogenemia
- Disseminated intravascular coagulation (DIC), as from obstetric-related causes, surgery, malignancy
- Fibrinolysis
- Artifactitious decrease due to diminished fibrin formation in the in vitro assay
- Severe liver disease
- Severe cachectic state
- Acquired dysfibrinogenemia during asparaginase therapy

## DECISION LEVELS          ACTIONS

| 30 mg/dl |

Spontaneous hemorrhage could occur when plasma fibrinogen is below this level. An appropriate therapeutic regimen should be initiated.

| 100 mg/dl |

Values below this level are consistent with diagnosis of DIC. Additional supporting information includes decreased platelet count and prolonged prothrombin time (PT). In addition, Factors V and VIII should be decreased.

| 500 mg/dl |

Values above this level are most often associated with one or more of the pathological conditions listed here. Additional diagnostic tests should be ordered.

# FOLATE IN SERUM

## Reference (normal) interval

**2–15 ng/ml
(4.4–33 nmol/L)**

Folate value is very assay-dependent.

## Causes of increased values

- Pernicious anemia
  (occasionally)

## Causes of decreased values

- Nutritional
- Malabsorption
- Hemolytic anemias
- Pregnancy
- Infancy
- Malignancies
- Drugs (phenobarbital,
  diphenylhydantoin, oral con-
  traceptives, methotrexate)

## DECISION LEVELS    ACTIONS

| 1.5 ng/ml | Values below this level are most always consistent with folate deficiency in a patient with megaloblastic anemia and a normal serum $B_{12}$. Appropriate therapy should be given. |

| 4.0 ng/ml | Values above 1.5 ng/ml but below this level are in the gray zone. If the diagnosis of folate deficiency is still suspected, a red blood cell folate should be ordered. A low RBC folate ($< 100$ $\mu g/L$) is confirmation of folic acid deficiency. |

# HEMATOCRIT

## Reference (normal) interval

0.38–0.46 L/L (adult females)
0.43–0.51 L/L (adult males)

## Causes of increased values

Relative polycythemia
• Stress
• Dehydration
• Diuretic therapy
• Burns
Absolute polycythemia
  *Primary (vera)*
  *Secondary*
• High altitude
• Impaired ventilation
• Cardiovascular disorders
• Impaired hemoglobin function
• Malignancy
• Benign tumors
• Renal disorders

## Causes of decreased values

With increased reticulocytes
• Hemolytic anemias, as from immunological causes, trauma on cells, abnormalities of the RBC membrane, hemoglobinopathies, or enzyme deficiencies
With decreased reticulocytes
  *Hypochromic microcytic anemia*
• Iron deficiency
• Thalassemia
• Anemia of chronic disease
• Sideroblastic anemia
  *Macrocytic anemia*
• Deficiency of vitamin $B_{12}$ or folate
• Effect of chemotherapy
  *Normochromic normocytic anemia*
• Marrow depression or failure

| | |
|---|---|
| 0.14 L/L | Values below this level would strongly suggest giving a therapeutic transfusion. However, the clinical setting should guide this decision, e.g., it may *not* be recommended if patient has congestive heart failure. |
| 0.33 L/L | Values below this level suggest a workup for causes of the anemia. RBC indices show what kind of anemia it is. Serum iron, $B_{12}$, and/or folate tests should be ordered, based on observing the blood smear and assessing the RBC indices and if reticulocytes are decreased. Monitor for changes in hematocrit values post-therapy. |
| 0.53 L/L in females<br>0.56 L/L in males | In addition to tests indicated when hemoglobin is over 17 g/dl (female) or over 18 g/dl (male), an assessment of plasma volume should be made when hematocrit is above these levels, so as to rule out relative polycythemia, which should *not* be treated by phlebotomy. |
| 0.70 L/L | Phlebotomy is urgently indicated when the values are at this level or above, as long as the diagnosis is either polycythemia vera or secondary polycythemia. |

# HEMOGLOBIN

## Reference (normal) interval

12–15.6 g/dl (adult females)
(120–156 g/L)

14–17.8 g/dl (adult males)
(140–178 g/L)

### Causes of increased values

Relative polycythemia
• Stress
• Dehydration
• Diuretic therapy
• Burns
Absolute polycythemia
*Primary (vera)*
*Secondary*
• High altitude
• Impaired ventilation
• Cardiovascular disorders
• Impaired hemoglobin function
• Malignancy
• Benign tumors
• Renal disorders

### Causes of decreased values

With increased reticulocytes
• Hemolytic anemias, as from immunological causes, trauma on cells, abnormalities of the RBC membrane, hemoglobinopathies, or enzyme deficiencies
With decreased reticulocytes
*Hypochromic microcytic anemia*
• Iron deficiency
• Thalassemia
• Anemia of chronic disease
• Sideroblastic anemia
*Macrocytic anemia*
• Deficiency of vitamin $B_{12}$ or folate
• Effect of chemotherapy
*Normochromic normocytic anemia*
• Marrow depression or failure

## DECISION LEVELS          ACTIONS

| 4.5 g/dl | Values lower than this level would strongly suggest giving a therapeutic transfusion. However, the clinical setting should guide this decision, e.g., it may *not* be recommended if patient has congestive heart failure. |

| 10.5 g/dl | Values below this level suggest a workup for causes of the anemia. RBC indices show what kind of anemia it is. Serum iron, $B_{12}$, and folate tests should be ordered, based on observing the blood smear and assessing the RBC indices and if reticulocytes are decreased. Monitor for changes in hemoglobin values post-therapy. |

| 17 g/dl in females 18 g/dl in males | Values above these levels suggest additional laboratory testing, i.e., WBC count, platelet count, leukocyte count, alkaline phosphatase, serum $B_{12}$ and unsaturated $B_{12}$ binding capacity, and $pO_2$ values, to classify the patient correctly. Phlebotomy is suggested in the symptomatic patient. |

| 23 g/dl | Treatment consisting of phlebotomy is urgently indicated when the values are at this level or above as long as the diagnosis is either polycythemia vera or secondary polycythemia. |

# MEAN CORPUSCULAR VOLUME (MCV)

## Reference (normal) interval

84–96 fl (cu $\mu$)

## Causes of increased values

- Megaloblastic anemia, as in vitamin $B_{12}$ deficiency, folate deficiency
- Liver disease
- Hypothyroidism
- Reticulocytosis
- Smoking
- History of ethanol abuse

## Causes of decreased values

- Iron deficiency anemia
- Thalassemia
- Anemia of chronic disease
- Sideroblastic anemia

## DECISION LEVELS    ACTIONS

| 80 fl |
|---|

In a patient with anemia and MCV lower than this level, additional testing, i.e., serum iron, IBC, and/or ferritin, should be done to confirm the diagnosis of iron deficiency anemia. If confirmed, then iron therapy should be administered and hemoglobin values monitored. The diagnosis of thalassemia is confirmed via hemoglobin electrophoresis with a quantitative analysis of $A_2$ and F hemoglobins.

| 100 fl |
|---|

In patients with anemia and MCV higher than this level, additional testing consisting of serum $B_{12}$, folate, and free $T_4$ index should be ordered to assist in their management.

# PARTIAL THROMBOPLASTIN TIME (PTT)

## Reference (normal) interval

Healthy subjects approximate the control value. Control value depends upon activator used in the assay. We assume control of 30 seconds.

## Causes of shortened values

## Causes of prolonged values

- Deficiency of fibrinogen
- Factor II deficiency
- Factor V deficiency
- Factor VIII deficiency
- Factor IX deficiency
- Factor X deficiency
- Factor XI deficiency
- Factor XII deficiency
- Fletcher trait (plasma prekalli-krein) deficiency
- Circulating antibodies (in-hibitors) to VII, IX
- Heparin therapy
- Liver disease
- Disseminated intravascular coagulation (DIC)

| DECISION LEVELS | ACTIONS |

| 35 seconds | If PTT is above this level, the patient should be evaluated for liver disease, factor deficiency, and circulating inhibitor. Tests include serum bilirubin, serum albumin, PT, PTT after mixing with normal plasma, and factor analyses. |

| 45 seconds | If patient is on heparin and the PTT is below this level, the dosage should be increased accordingly. |

| 90 seconds | If patient is on heparin and the PTT is above this level, the dosage should be decreased to avoid spontaneous hemorrhage. The decision level chosen is still one of controversy. |

# PLASMINOGEN

## Reference (normal) interval

80–120% of normal human pooled plasma (NHPP)

## Causes of increased values

- Pregnancy
- Inflammation
- Myocardial infarction
- Bacterial infection

## Causes of decreased values

- Disseminated intravascular coagulation (DIC)
- Thrombolytic therapy
- Thrombosis
- Liver disease
- Hereditary deficiencies
- Surgery/trauma

| DECISION LEVELS | ACTIONS |

| 50% of NHPP | Values below this level definitely indicate plasminogen deficiency. The combination of decreased AT III, Factors V and VIII, platelets, and fibrinogen would confirm the diagnosis of DIC. |

| 75% of NHPP | Values below this level suggest a number of pathological causes. Appropriate confirmation should be sought through additional laboratory testing. |

| 135% of NHPP | Values above this level in the nonpregnant female suggest inflammation. This can be confirmed with additional laboratory data. |

# PLATELET COUNT

## Reference (normal) interval

150,000–400,000/$\mu$l
(150 x 10$^9$–400 x 10$^9$/L)

## Causes of increased values

- Splenectomy
- Malignancy
- Myeloproliferative disease, such as polycythemia vera, chronic myelogenous leukemia
- Infection
- Acute blood loss (iron deficiency)
- Inflammatory bowel disease
- Collagen-vascular disorder

## Causes of decreased values

- Production failure, as in megakaryocytopenia, aplastic anemia, displacement, ineffective thrombopoiesis
- Immune destruction – idiopathic thrombocytopenic purpura (ITP), post-transfusion, drug-induced
- Mechanical destruction (splenomegaly), as in Banti's syndrome, Felty's syndrome, lupus erythematosus, Gaucher's disease, myeloproliferative syndrome, lymphoma
- Increased utilization (coagulopathy), as in disseminated intravascular coagulation (DIC), hemolytic-uremic syndrome (HUS), thrombotic thrombocytopenic purpura (TTP)
- Massive transfusion (i.e., dilutional)
- Familial causes: Wiskott-Aldrich syndrome, May-Hegglin anomaly, thrombopoietin deficiency, thrombocytopenia with absent radius (TAR), giant platelet syndrome

## DECISION LEVELS · ACTIONS

| 10,000/$\mu$l | Spontaneous hemorrhage may develop when the platelet count is lower than this level. With a bleeding time of 15 min or more and/or in the presence of bleeding, therapeutic measures in the form of platelet concentrates should be administered. |

| 50,000/$\mu$l | If patient demonstrates minor bleeding lesions or will undergo minor surgery and the platelet count is lower than this level, then platelet concentrates should be given. |

| 100,000/$\mu$l | If patient demonstrates major bleeding lesions or will undergo major surgery and the platelet count is lower than this level, then platelet concentrates should be given. |

| 600,000/$\mu$l | Values above this level suggest pathology. In the absence of a history of blood loss or splenectomy, a careful search for malignancy should be made. |

| 1,000,000/$\mu$l | Values above this level often result in thrombosis. Antiplatelet drugs should be given if the thrombocytosis is more than transient in nature. |

# PROTHROMBIN TIME (PT)

## Reference (normal) interval

We assume a control of 11.5 seconds.
Healthy subjects should approximate the control ($\pm 2$ seconds).

## Causes of shortened values   Causes of prolonged values

- Factor II deficiency
- Factor V deficiency
- Factor VII deficiency
- Factor X deficiency
- Warfarin therapy
- Liver insufficiency
- Vitamin K deficiency
- In vivo inhibitors
- Poor fat absorption
- Hypofibrinogenemia
- Disseminated intravascular coagulation (DIC)

**14 seconds**

A value above this level in a patient known to have liver disease signifies less than 50% of the associated factor present. Factor assays and PTT should be performed, as well as a test for circulating inhibitor.

**16 seconds**

A value below this level in a patient who is on warfarin would suggest inadequate anticoagulation. Dosage should be increased. Values at this level or higher in a patient who is to undergo major surgery would suggest correctional therapy.

**30 seconds**

A value above this level in a patient on warfarin suggests excessive anticoagulation. Dosage should be reduced.

# VITAMIN B$_{12}$ IN SERUM

## Reference (normal) interval

200–900 pg/ml
(150–670 pmol/L)

## Causes of increased values

- Leukemia, especially in myelocytic leukemia, but also in 33% of cases of lymphocytic leukemia
- Polycythemia vera
- Hepatitis (acute and chronic)
- Hepatic encephalopathy
- Hepatic cirrhosis

## Causes of decreased values

- Pernicious anemia (lack of intrinsic factor)
- Gastrectomy
- Resected or diseased ileum, e.g., celiaca, Crohn's disease, regional enteritis
- Transcobalamin deficiency
- Blind loop syndrome
- Fish tapeworm infestation
- Extreme vegetarian diets
- Primary hypothyroidism
- Pregnancy
- Inadequate dietary intake

| 170 pg/ml |
| :---: |

Values below this level are often consistent with vitamin $B_{12}$ deficiency. To confirm the diagnosis of pernicious anemia, additional testing for intrinsic factor blocking, antibody, serum gastrin or the more definitive Schilling test is recommended in the patient with megaloblastic anemia and a depressed $B_{12}$ value.

| 250 pg/ml |
| :---: |

Values above this level tend to rule out vitamin $B_{12}$ deficiency as cause of the anemia. Serum folate and bone marrow examinations may be appropriate if the diagnosis is in doubt in a patient with macrocytic anemia.

| 1200 pg/ml |
| :---: |

Values above this level suggest various pathologies. An examination of the peripheral blood smear is appropriate to rule out polycythemia vera or leukemia as the associated pathological process.

# WHITE BLOOD CELL COUNT

## Reference (normal) interval

4000–10,000/$\mu$l
(4 x 10$^9$–10 x 10$^9$/L)

## Causes of increased values

- Physiologic, as with severe exercise, hypoxia, stress, injection with epinephrine
- Infection, especially bacterial
- Toxic states, e.g., uremia, eclampsia, gout, diabetic acidosis, or from drugs or chemicals
- Tissue destruction, as with myocardial infarction, burns, surgery, crush injuries
- Nonhematologic malignancy
- Hemorrhage
- Hemolysis
- Leukemia
- Splenectomy
- Infectious mononucleosis

## Causes of decreased values

- Infection, e.g., typhoid fever, paratyphoid fever, brucellosis
- Drugs, e.g., chloramphenicol
- Megaloblastic anemia
- Splenomegaly, as with congestive splenomegaly, Felty's syndrome, Gaucher's disease, lymphoma, Niemann-Pick disease
- Systemic lupus erythematosus
- Aplastic anemia

## DECISION LEVELS    ACTIONS

| 500/$\mu$l |
|---|

Values below this level denote a great risk of infection in the patient. Appropriate preventive measures, as well as careful monitoring for infection, should be instituted.

| 3000/$\mu$l |
|---|

Values below this level are consistent with leukopenia. Additional diagnostic testing— WBC differential count, observation of the peripheral blood smear, and drug-intake history—should be done.

| 12,000/$\mu$l |
|---|

Values above this level are consistent with leukocytosis. The differential count would be of value to characterize the cause and the type of the increased WBC. A source of infection should be sought, if appropriate.

| 30,000/$\mu$l |
|---|

Values above this level suggest the possibility of leukemia. Differential count, observation of the peripheral smear, and bone marrow examination might be considered.

| |
|---|

# 6

# Miscellaneous Tests

# FOAM STABILITY INDEX (FSI)
# IN AMNIOTIC FLUID

## Reference (normal) interval

Mature specimens usually $\geq 47$

## Causes of increased values

- Mature lungs in the fetus
- Contamination with blood and/or meconium

## Causes of decreased values

- Immature lungs in the fetus

## DECISION LEVELS          ACTIONS

| | |
|---|---|
| **44** | Values at this level and lower are often associated with the respiratory distress syndrome (RDS). If possible, delivery should be postponed until the value becomes mature. |

| | |
|---|---|
| **47** | Values at this level and above are almost always associated with mature lungs. In the absence of blood and/or meconium contamination, such values suggest that delivery of the baby would be appropriate if there are other clinical reasons to deliver. |

# LECITHIN/SPHINGOMYELIN (L/S) RATIO IN AMNIOTIC FLUID

## Reference (normal) interval

Mature specimens usually $\geq 2.0$

## Causes of increased values

- Mature lungs in the fetus
- Maternal diabetes and fetal pulmonary immaturity
- Contamination with blood and/or meconium

## Causes of decreased values

- Immature lungs in the fetus
- Intrauterine growth retardation in the small-for-gestational-age (SGA) baby with mature lungs

## DECISION LEVELS ACTIONS

| 1.5 | Values at this level and lower are often associated with the respiratory distress syndrome (RDS). If possible, delivery should be postponed until the value becomes mature. Other testing, e.g., FSI and phosphatidyl glycerol (PG), is suggested. |

| 2.0 | Values at this level and above are usually associated with mature lungs. However, maternal diabetes and subsequent RDS may be associated with such values. |

| 3.0 | Values at this level and above are almost always associated with mature lungs. In the absence of blood and/or meconium contamination, such values suggest that delivery of the baby would be advisable if there are other clinical reasons to deliver. |

# RED BLOOD CELLS IN URINE SEDIMENT

## Reference (normal) interval

1–2/high-power field

## Causes of increased values    Causes of decreased values

- Cystitis
- Bladder tumor
- Trigonitis
- Benign prostatic hyperplasia
- Prostatitis
- Prostatic cancer
- Varices of bladder
- Varices of prostate
- Renal neoplasm
- Glomerulonephritis
- Renal stone
- Pyelonephritis
- Trauma
- Urethritis
- Urethral stricture
- Urethral diverticulum
- Tuberculosis
- Generalized bleeding disorder
- Essential hematuria
- Congenital anomalies
- Fever
- Prolonged heavy exercise

## DECISION LEVELS    ACTIONS

| 1/high-power field | Values of 0–1 RBC/hpf are acceptable. In the absence of pathologic signs in the history, physical examination, or urinalysis, no other tests are necessary. |

| 5/high-power field | In the absence of gross hematuria, a value at this level or higher suggests urine culture and susceptibility (25% of cases have urethritis). In a male, careful examination of the prostate is recommended. Urine should be observed for the presence of RBCs or heme-pigmented granular casts, which supports the diagnosis of glomerular disease. Persistent, undiagnosed microscopic hematuria, even if it is asymptomatic, demands an intravenous urogram. |

| Gross hematuria | If gross hematuria is confirmed by the presence of RBCs in the sediment, the most likely diagnoses in adults are cystitis (in 25% of cases) and carcinoma of bladder or kidney (in 17% of cases). Urine culture and susceptibility should be ordered to confirm the diagnosis of infection, and if it is positive, appropriate antibiotic therapy should be given. If testing is negative, an intravenous urogram is indicated to assess the kidneys, renal pelves, and ureters for any lesions. Prostate should also be palpated. |

# URINARY PROTEIN

## Reference (normal) interval

0–150 mg/24 hours

## Causes of increased values   Causes of decreased values

- Severe muscular exertion
- Pregnancy (slight proteinuria)
- Preeclampsia of pregnancy (massive proteinuria)
- Orthostatic (postural) proteinuria (slight proteinuria)
- Febrile proteinuria (mild proteinuria)
- Venous congestion, as with renal vein thrombosis
- Arteriosclerotic renal vascular disease
- Arterial hypertension
- Congestive heart failure
- Pyelonephritis
- Polycystic renal disease
- Glomerulonephritis—acute, subacute, or chronic
- Membranous glomerulonephritis (often massive proteinuria)
- Drug-induced nephrotoxins, e.g., mercury, carbon tetrachloride
- Lipoid nephrosis (often massive proteinuria)
- Kimmelstiel-Wilson syndrome
- Polyarteritis nodosa
- Multiple myeloma
- Amyloidosis
- Diabetic benign nephrosclerosis

| 500 mg/24 hours |
|---|

Persistent proteinuria greater than this level is strong evidence of renal disease. After benign causes are excluded, a diagnostic renal biopsy should be considered.

| 3000 mg/24 hours |
|---|

A value at this level or higher in association with edema and hypoalbuminemia is consistent with the diagnosis of nephrotic syndrome. In a pregnant patient with hypertension, the diagnosis is preeclampsia. The latter case demands careful monitoring of fetus, assessing maternal hemostatic balance, and watching for convulsions.

| 8000 mg/24 hours |
|---|

A value at this level or higher suggests massive protein loss. Based on the results of renal biopsy, steroid therapy may be recommended. In a crisis, intravenous albumin may be of symptomatic benefit.

# WHITE BLOOD CELLS IN URINE SEDIMENT

## Reference (normal) interval

1–2/high-power field (males)
1–5/high-power field (females)

## Causes of increased values    Causes of decreased values

- Urinary tract infection
Sterile pyuria
- Prostatitis—chlamydial, viral, or mycoplasmal in younger patients; from bacterial colonization or infection in older patients
- Acute urethritis—chlamydial, monilial, trichomonal, or from trauma, foreign bodies
- Urinary tract tuberculosis
(See also causes of increased values under Red Blood Cells in Urine Sediment, page 134.)

| DECISION LEVELS | ACTIONS |
|---|---|
| 1/high-power field | Values of 0–1 WBC/hpf in a specimen with no protein, no RBCs, and no casts present would tend to rule out a urinary tract infection. Order a urine culture and susceptibility only if the clinical picture demands it. |
| 5/high-power field | Values at this level or higher in an appropriately collected urine specimen would strongly suggest sending the urine for culture and susceptibility. |
| 50/high-power field | Values at this level or higher not explained by gross hematuria most often represent bacterial infection. Aggressive diagnostic and therapeutic maneuvers should be started. |

# Drugs

# AMIKACIN (AMIKIN)

## Indications

- Antibiotic therapy

## Therapeutic range

20–30 $\mu$g/ml (peak)
1–8 $\mu$g/ml (trough)

## Symptoms of toxicity

- Ototoxicity
- Nephrotoxicity

| DECISION LEVELS | ACTIONS |
|---|---|
| 10 μg/ml (trough) | If sustained trough value is higher than this level, side effects may occur. Dosage should be decreased and renal function monitored. |
| 20 μg/ml (peak) | If peak value is below this level, dosage should be increased to reach therapeutic interval. Repeat testing is recommended. |
| 32 μg/ml (peak) | If peak value is higher than this level, ototoxicity or nephrotoxicity may occur. Dosage should be decreased and renal function should be monitored. |

# CARBAMAZEPINE (TEGRETOL)

## Indications

- Antiepileptic for tonoclonic (grand mal) seizures and complex partial seizures
- Analgesic for trigeminal neuralgia

## Therapeutic range

4–12 μg/ml (17–51 μmol/L)
4–8 μg/ml in patients receiving multiple antiepileptics
8–12 μg/ml in patients taking only this drug

## Symptoms of toxicity

- Dizziness
- Incoordination
- Diplopia
- Drowsiness
- Nausea and vomiting

## DECISION LEVELS      ACTIONS

| 4 μg/ml | If value is below this level, the dosage of drug should be increased to reach the therapeutic interval. |

| 9 μg/ml | If patient is on other antiepileptic drugs, toxicity may occur. The dosage should be regulated to get back into the appropriate therapeutic interval. |

| 14 μg/ml | Toxic symptoms are seen when values are above this level, even if the patient is on no other antiepileptic drug. The clinical status of the patient should be reassessed with respect to therapeutic goals. If necessary, the dosage should be reduced to get back into the appropriate therapeutic interval. |

## DIGOXIN (LANOXIN)

### Indications

- Treatment of congestive heart failure
- Management of supraventricular tachyarrhythmias

### Therapeutic range

0.9–2.0 ng/ml
(1.15–2.56 nmol/L)

### Symptoms of toxicity

- Anorexia
- Nausea and vomiting
- Diarrhea
- Abdominal pain
- Headache
- Fatigue
- Malaise
- Drowsiness
- Blurring of vision
- Diplopia
- Extrasystole
- AV block
- Sinus arrhythmia
- Paroxysmal tachycardia
- Atrial fibrillation
- Ventricular fibrillation

## DECISION LEVELS          ACTIONS

| 1.0 ng/ml | Values below this level may represent noncompliance. In the nonresponder, dosage should be raised until either signs of toxicity occur or upper therapeutic level is reached. |

| 1.6 ng/ml | In the presence of symptoms of drug toxicity, values above this level would suggest decreasing dosage. |

| 2.5 ng/ml | Serious toxic effects, including cardiac effects, are noted often with values above this level. The dosage should be reduced dramatically. |

# DISOPYRAMIDE (NORPACE)

## Indications

• Suppression and prevention of ventricular arrhythmias

## Therapeutic range

2.5–5.0 μg/ml
(7.5–15.0 μmol/L)

## Symptoms of toxicity

Anticholinergic side effects
• Dry mouth
• Urinary hesitancy
• Constipation
• Urinary obstruction
Cardiac effects
• Widening of QRS interval
• Congestive heart failure
• Hypotension
• Various conduction
  disturbances
• Bradycardia
• Asystole

## DECISION LEVELS          ACTIONS

| 2.5 µg/ml | If value is below this level, the dosage should be increased to reach the therapeutic range. |

| 4.5 µg/ml | Values above this level may be associated with various anticholinergic side effects. Such side effects suggest lowering dosage and/or considering alternative therapy. |

| 7.0 µg/ml | Values above this level may be associated with serious toxicities. The dosage should be lowered. In case of overdose and values above this level in the presence of serious cardiac side effects, inotropic agents such as isoproterenol are suggested, as well as hemodialysis. |

# ETHOSUXIMIDE (ZARONTIN)

## Indications

• Antiepileptic for absence (petit mal) seizures

## Therapeutic range

**50–100 μg/ml**
**(355–710 μmol/L)**

## Symptoms of toxicity

• Gastric distress
• Nausea and vomiting
• Anorexia
• Fatigue
• Lethargy
• Headache
• Dizziness

**Note:** Toxicity does <u>not</u> correlate well with blood levels.

50 $\mu$g/ml

With values below this level, the dosage of the drug should be increased to reach the therapeutic range.

120 $\mu$g/ml

If the value is below this level and the patient continues to have absence seizures, additional dosage can be given. With values above this level, the clinical status of the patient should be reassessed with respect to therapeutic goals. If necessary, consider alternative therapy.

# GENTAMICIN (GARAMYCIN)

## Indications

• Antibiotic therapy

## Therapeutic range

6–10 $\mu$g/ml (peak)
0.5–1.5 $\mu$g/ml (trough)

## Symptoms of toxicity

• Ototoxicity
• Nephrotoxicity

| DECISION LEVELS | ACTIONS |
|---|---|

| 0.5 µg/ml (trough) | If trough value is below this level, dosage should be increased to reach therapeutic interval. Repeat testing is recommended. |

| 2 µg/ml (trough) | If sustained trough value is above this level, side effects may occur. Dosage should be decreased and renal function should be monitored. |

| 6 µg/ml (peak) | If peak value is below this level, dosage should be increased to reach therapeutic interval. Repeat testing is recommended. |

| 12 µg/ml (peak) | If peak value is above this level, ototoxicity or nephrotoxicity may occur. Dosage should be decreased and renal function should be monitored. |

# KANAMYCIN (KANTREX)

## Indications

• Antibiotic therapy

## Therapeutic range

20–30 $\mu$g/ml (peak)
1–8 $\mu$g/ml (trough)

## Symptoms of toxicity

• Ototoxicity
• Nephrotoxicity

| DECISION LEVELS | ACTIONS |
|---|---|
| 10 μg/ml (trough) | If sustained trough value is above this level, side effects may occur. Dosage should be decreased and renal function monitored. |
| 20 μg/ml (peak) | If peak value is below this level, dosage should be increased to reach therapeutic interval. Repeat testing is recommended. |
| 32 μg/ml (peak) | If peak value is above this level, ototoxicity or nephrotoxicity may occur. Dosage should be decreased and renal function should be monitored. |

## LIDOCAINE (ANESTACON, XYLOCAINE)

### Indications

- Ventricular arrhythmias associated with acute myocardial infarction, cardiac manipulation, or digitalis toxicity

### Therapeutic range

**1.5–5.0 $\mu$g/ml**
**(6 to 21 $\mu$mol/L)**

### Symptoms of toxicity

- Drowsiness
- Paresthesias
- Dizziness
- Convulsions
- Coma
- Sinus bradycardia
- Complete heart block

| DECISION LEVELS | ACTIONS |

| 1.5 µg/ml | If value is below this level in a patient who continues to have arrhythmias, the dosage should be increased to reach the therapeutic range. |

| 5.0 µg/ml | If value is equal to or above this level, therapy should be modified to decrease likelihood of drug toxicity. |

| 7.0 µg/ml | When value is above this level, the dosage should be decreased before toxicity occurs. |

**Note:** Pharmacological activity of lidocaine is directly related to the free drug concentrations because plasma concentrations of lidocaine-binding protein may be elevated in patients under stress, as in myocardial infarction. The free lidocaine concentration may be within the therapeutic range, even though the total plasma lidocaine concentration may be elevated. Therefore, the clinical status of the patient must be monitored carefully when interpreting lidocaine concentration.

# LITHIUM

## Indications

- Psychiatric disorders

## Therapeutic range

0.5–1.2 mmol/L

## Symptoms of toxicity

- Hand tremors
- Polyuria
- Goiter
- Weight gain

## Causes of increased values    Causes of decreased values

- Lithium medication given in
  excessive amounts

| DECISION LEVELS | ACTIONS |
|---|---|

| 0.4 mmol/L | A value at this level or lower signifies that the patient is not receiving an adequate amount of drug. Consider increasing the dosage if the clinical symptoms warrant. |

| 0.8 mmol/L | A value at this level is well within the therapeutic range. If the patient is not responding, consider alternative therapies. |

| 1.5 mmol/L | A value at this level or greater is above the therapeutic interval and could result in drug toxicity. Consider decreasing the dosage. |

# PHENOBARBITAL (LUMINAL)

## Indications

- All seizure disorders, except absence (petit mal) seizures
- Status epilepticus and febrile seizures

## Therapeutic range

**15–40 $\mu$g/ml**
**(65–172 $\mu$mol/L)**

## Symptoms of toxicity

- Sedation (most common)
- Lethargy
- Stupor
- Impaired cognitive function
- Coma

## DECISION LEVELS    ACTIONS

| 15 $\mu$g/ml |
| --- |

If value is below this level, the dosage of the drug should be increased to reach the therapeutic interval.

| 30 $\mu$g/ml |
| --- |

If value is below this level and patient continues to have seizures, additional dosage can be given. When value is above this level, consider alternative or combined therapy.

| 60 $\mu$g/ml |
| --- |

When value is above this level, reduce dosage of drug. Values above this level are usually associated with serious toxic effects such as lethargy, stupor, impaired cognitive function, and coma.

| 120 $\mu$g/ml |
| --- |

When value is above this level, patient will be toxic. Give CNS, cardiac, and respiratory support as needed.

## PHENYTOIN (DILANTIN)

### Indications

- All seizure disorders, except absence (petit mal) seizures

### Therapeutic range

10–20 µg/ml
(39–79 µmol/L)

### Symptoms of toxicity

- Nystagmus
- Blurred vision
- Ataxia
- Dysarthria
- Drowsiness
- Respiratory distress
- Confusion
- Irritability
- Hallucinations
- Delusions
- Coma

| DECISION LEVELS | ACTIONS |
|---|---|

| 10 $\mu$g/ml | If value is below this level and if no other antiepileptic is given in combined therapy, it is advisable to increase dosage to reach the therapeutic range. |

| 20 $\mu$g/ml | If value is above this level, decrease dosage, because toxic effects are very likely to occur. |

| 50 $\mu$g/ml | If value of patient in respiratory distress is above this level, consider active support. |

## PRIMIDONE (MYSOLINE)

### Indications

• Major motor, elementary, and complex partial seizures

### Therapeutic range

5 to 12 $\mu$g/ml
(23–55 $\mu$mol/L)

### Symptoms of toxicity

• Sedation (most common)
• Nausea and vomiting
• Diplopia
• Dizziness
• Ataxia

**Note:** Side effects are usually plasma-level related. Phenobarbital concentration should also be taken into account because it is a major metabolite of primidone.

| | |
|---|---|
| 5 μg/ml | If value is below this level, the dosage of the drug should be increased to reach the therapeutic interval. |
| 9 μg/ml | If value is below this level and patient continues to have seizures and there are no side effects (ataxia or lethargy), additional dosage can be given. If value is above this level, consider alternative or combined therapy. |
| 12 μg/ml | When value is above this level, the clinical status of the patient should be reassessed with respect to therapeutic goals. If necessary, reduce the dosage. Values above this level are most often associated with sedation, nausea, ataxia, and dizziness. |

## PROCAINAMIDE (PRONESTYL)

### Indications

- Treatment of premature ventricular contractions, ventricular tachycardia, atrial fibrillations, and paroxysmal atrial tachycardia

### Therapeutic range

4–10 $\mu$g/ml
(15 to 37 $\mu$mol/L)

10–30 $\mu$g/ml
(for sum of procainamide and N-acetyl-procainamide)

### Symptoms of toxicity

- Cardiac effects, i.e., bradycardia, hypotension, prolongation of ECG intervals, arrhythmias, myocardial depression
- Sweating
- Disorientation
- Nausea and vomiting
- Malaise
- Systemic lupus erythematosus in approximately 30 percent of patients on chronic therapy

| | |
|---|---|
| 4 $\mu$g/ml <br> 10 $\mu$g/ml* | With values below these levels, the dosage of the drug should be increased to reach the therapeutic range. |
| 12 $\mu$g/ml <br> 30 $\mu$g/ml* | If values are at these levels and patient has not responded, alternative therapy should be administered. |
| 16 $\mu$g/ml <br> 40 $\mu$g/ml* | With values at these levels or higher, the dosage should be decreased to avoid drug toxicity. |

*For sum of procainamide and N-acetyl-procainamide.

# QUINIDINE

## Indications

- Prevention and treatment of supraventricular arrhythmias
- Prevention and treatment of ventricular arrhythmias

## Therapeutic range

2–5 $\mu$g/ml
(6–15 $\mu$mol/L)

## Symptoms of toxicity

- Hypotension
- QRS widening
- Heart block
- Cinchonism (headache, dizziness, tinnitus, nervousness, blurred vision, nausea, and vomiting)
- Nausea
- Diarrhea

## DECISION LEVELS          ACTIONS

| 2 $\mu$g/ml |
|---|

If value is below this level, dosage of the drug should be increased to reach the therapeutic range.

| 5 $\mu$g/ml |
|---|

If value is at this level or higher and patient has not responded adequately, alternative therapy should be instituted.

| 7 $\mu$g/ml |
|---|

When value is above this level, dosage should be decreased to prevent drug toxicity.

# SALICYLATES

## Indications

- Treatment of rheumatic diseases
- Treatment of chronic inflammatory diseases

## Therapeutic range

150–300 $\mu$g/ml
(15–30 mg/dl)
(1.1–2.2 mmol/L)

## Symptoms of toxicity

- Tinnitus
- Dizziness
- Depression of auditory and visual acuity
- Sweating
- Nausea and vomiting
- Respiratory alkalosis (early)
- Metabolic acidosis (late)
- Confusion
- Convulsions
- Coma

## DECISION LEVELS  ACTIONS

| 150 $\mu$g/ml |
|---|

A value below this level in a patient treated for rheumatic disease may represent noncompliance or inadequate dosing. Dosage should be increased to reach the therapeutic range.

| 300 $\mu$g/ml |
|---|

Values above this level are associated with mild toxicity, e.g., tinnitus, dizziness. If such symptoms occur, the dosage should be decreased.

| 500 $\mu$g/ml |
|---|

Values above this level are often associated with severe toxicity, e.g., irrationality, confusion, convulsions, coma. Appropriate supportive measures should be instituted. Acute overdose would indicate gastric lavage as well as alkalization of the urine.

# THEOPHYLLINE

## Indications

- Treatment of asthma and chronic obstructive pulmonary disease
- Treatment of neonatal apnea

## Therapeutic range

10–20 $\mu$g/ml for asthma
(55–111 $\mu$mol/L)

5–10 $\mu$g/ml for neonatal apnea
(28-55 $\mu$mol/L)

## Symptoms of toxicity

- Nausea and vomiting
- Diarrhea
- Headache
- Irritability
- Cardiac arrhythmias
- Seizures

| DECISION LEVELS | ACTIONS |
|---|---|

| | |
|---|---|
| 10 μg/ml | If value is below this level, the patient may not be compliant or the dosage is too low. The noncompliant patient should be encouraged to take the drug. The dosage should be modified until the concentration is in the therapeutic interval. |
| 20 μg/ml | Values above this level may be associated with toxic side effects. In case of symptoms of drug toxicity and a value higher than this level, the dosage should be decreased until the symptoms cease. |
| 35 μg/ml | Values above this level are often associated with serious side effects, including death. The patient should be carefully monitored. Seizures can occur with values lower than 30 μg/ml. |
| 60 μg/ml | When the serum concentration is above this level, charcoal hemoperfusion should be considered to rapidly remove theophylline and prevent seizures. |

## TOBRAMYCIN (NEBCIN)

### Indications

• Antibiotic therapy

### Therapeutic range

6–10 $\mu$g/ml (peak)
0.5–1.5 $\mu$g/ml (trough)

### Symptoms of toxicity

• Ototoxicity
• Nephrotoxicity

## DECISION LEVELS    ACTIONS

| 0.5 μg/ml (trough) | If trough value is below this level, dosage should be increased to reach therapeutic interval. Repeat testing is recommended. |

| 2 μg/ml (trough) | If sustained trough value is higher than this level, side effects may occur. Dosage should be decreased and renal function should be monitored. |

| 6 μg/ml (peak) | If peak value is below this level, dosage should be increased to reach therapeutic interval. Repeat testing is recommended. |

| 12 μg/ml (peak) | If peak value is over this level, ototoxicity or nephrotoxicity may occur. Dosage should be decreased and renal function should be monitored. |

## VALPROIC ACID (DEPAKENE)

### Indications

- Seizure disorders, including generalized absence, generalized tonoclonic, and partial seizures

### Therapeutic range

50–100 $\mu$g/ml
(347–693 $\mu$mol/L)

### Symptoms of toxicity

- Nausea and vomiting
- Drowsiness
- Hepatotoxicity
- Acute toxic encephalopathy

## DECISION LEVELS    ACTIONS

| 50 μg/ml | If value is below this level, it is advisable to increase dosage to reach therapeutic range. |

| 90 μg/ml | If value is below this level and there is inadequate seizure control, dosage should be increased. Values above this level warrant monitoring for hepatotoxicity. |

| 120 μg/ml | If value is above this level, the clinical status of the patient should be reassessed with respect to therapeutic goals. Tests for hepatotoxicity, e.g., aminotransferase, fibrinogen, and alkaline phosphatase should be ordered. If necessary, decrease the dosage. Monitor for hepatotoxicity whenever giving this drug because the most severe hepatotoxicity may occur even though the valproic acid concentration is within the therapeutic range. |

# ALPHABETICAL INDEX OF ANALYTES

**Laboratory Diagnosis and Patient Monitoring: Clinical Chemistry**
Robert S. Galen, M.D., and Leslie Brennan, Editors
ISBN 0-87489-265-1

**Laboratory Diagnosis and Patient Monitoring: Immunology**
Robert S. Galen, M.D., and Leslie Brennan, Editors
ISBN 0-87489-365-9

**Patient Care FlowChart Manual, Third Edition**
ISBN 0-87489-295-3

**Human Disease in Color**
Chandler Smith, M.D.
ISBN 0-87489-188-4

**Core Pathology: Fundamental Concepts and Principles**
Chandler Smith, M.D.
ISBN 0-87489-239-2

**Physician's Guide to Oculosystemic Diseases**
William V. Delaney, M.D.
ISBN 0-87489-250-3

**Physician's Guide to Diseases of the Oral Cavity**
Harriet S. Goldman, D.D.S., M.P.H., and
Michael Z. Marder, D.D.S.
ISBN 0-87489-240-6

**Drug Interactions Index**
Fred Lerman, M.D., and Robert T. Weibert, Pharm.D.
ISBN 0-87489-266-X

## Isler's Pocket Dictionary of Diagnostic Tests, Procedures & Terms
Charlotte Isler, R.N.
ISBN 0-87489-189-2

## Laboratory Communication: Getting Your Message Through
Arthur F. Krieg, M.D.
ISBN 0-87489-185-X

## Managing the Patient-Focused Laboratory
George D. Lundberg, M.D., Editor
ISBN 0-87489-065-9

## Sharpening Laboratory Management Skills
Edward M. Friedman, Editor
ISBN 0-87489-204-X

## A Practical Guide to Financial Management of the Clinical Laboratory
Janiece Sattler
ISBN 0-87489-235-X

## Legal Guidelines for the Clinical Laboratory
Robert J. Fitzgibbon, Editor
ISBN 0-87489-243-0

## The Effective Laboratory Supervisor
William O. Umiker, M.D.
ISBN 0-87489-269-4

For information, write to
**MEDICAL ECONOMICS BOOKS**
Oradell, New Jersey 07649
Or call toll-free: 1-800-223-0581, ext. 2755
(Within the 201 area: 262-3030, ext. 2755)